ENTRY STRATEGIES
FOR SCHOOL CONSULTATION

The Guilford School Practitioner Series

EDITORS

STEPHEN N. ELLIOTT, Ph.D.
University of Wisconsin—Madison

JOSEPH C. WITT, Ph.D.
Louisiana State University, Baton Rouge

ENTRY STRATEGIES
FOR
SCHOOL CONSULTATION

EDWARD S. MARKS, Ph.D.

THE GUILFORD PRESS
New York   London

© 1995 The Guilford Press
A Division of Guilford Publications, Inc.
72 Spring Street, New York, NY 10012

Printed in the United States of America

This book is printed on acid-free paper.

Last digit is print number: 9 8 7 6 5 4 3 2 1

Library of Congress Cataloging-in-Publication Data

Marks, Edward S.
    Entry strategies for school consultation / by Edward S. Marks.
        p. cm.—(The Guilford school practitioner series)
    Includes bibliographical references (p.) and index.
    ISBN 0-89862-368-5
    1. Educational consultants—United States. 2. Educational counseling—United States. 3. School children—Mental health services—United States.   I. Title. II. Series.
LB2799.2.M36   1995   94-27760
371.7'13—dc20   CIP

To Sarah and Benjamin

*May better schools
with empowered staff
give you a brighter future.*

Preface

The need for "special services teams" to expand from traditional evaluation, classification, and placement of students in special education
classes to broader, preventive roles has been well-documented over the
past decade or more by Medway (1982) and others. In 1980, the Spring
Hill Symposium on School Psychology (sponsored by the U.S. Department of Education and the major psychology associations, at Spring
Hill, MN) set the tone for school psychologists to become more involved
with school administrators, teachers, policy, curriculum, parents, and
community. Moreover, the recommendations of this conference have
relevance to other consultants working inside the schools, such as school
social workers, guidance counselors, and remedial teachers or learning
disability specialists (referred to as special services personnel or teams),
as well as outside consultants such as university professors, mental health
specialists from clinics and hospitals, and teacher trainers.

Hence, this book reaches out to inside and outside consultants by
providing practical guidelines to accomplish the goals of entering a
school to do consultation. "Entry," as used here, is defined as follows:

1. Gaining access to building administrators, particularly principals,
   so that consultation efforts will be sanctioned.
2. Obtaining support of higher-level administration (at district
   level) to do consulting.
3. Utilizing the efforts of teachers, as well as all other building
   employees, to help make consultation work.
4. Overcoming resistance to consultation.

Who are consultants inside the school system? Most often they are
people already employed by the system, who offer their expertise to

improve education. Counselors, school psychologists, counseling psychologists, and educational psychologists consult with teachers to help them handle children more effectively and to make the curriculum more responsive to student needs and system demands. Guidance counselors work with teachers and administrators to apply career development concepts to school programs and to improve students' mental health.

Learning specialists, usually teachers with advanced degrees, knowledgeable in such areas as reading remediation, learning disabilities, and so forth, evaluate students' skills in reading, language, mathematics, and other academic areas; help other teachers with curriculum and remedial issues; or help administrators develop curriculum and decide on text purchases. These learning specialists may teach remedial classes themselves (resource rooms and Title I or basic skills reading and math programs); thus, they are more readily available to the regular classroom teacher than are outside consultants. The itinerant teacher, working with more than one school, also plays a consultant role and could find information of value here.

School social workers consult in the schools and often work with special teams to evaluate the impact of families on student performance. In this book they may find means to encourage administrators to be more responsive to family concerns. It is my hope that school social workers, using the techniques suggested here, will also find classroom consulting easier to accomplish.

Speech and language therapists often are part of school special services teams and consult with teachers to help meet the language development of students. They also need entry skills in order to be more effective.

Outside consultants are likely to be university professors carrying out projects on a larger scale (e.g., a statewide program in which learning specialists and regular education teachers consult to avoid removing students with remedial needs from the regular classroom) (Knight, Meyers, Paolucci-Whitcomb, Hasaszi, & Nevin, 1981). These outside consultants have less of a school constituency. They need entry skills because it is likely that the local school principal and teachers had little to do with developing their project. As researchers, they must go beyond their own project to view the school systemically.

Mental health personnel from community mental health centers, who consult with schools on developing emotionally healthy environments (Caplan, 1970) and who deal with classroom management problems, may find ideas here for effective outreach to staff.

Others who consult include school administrators who are curriculum, computer, or behavior specialists. They must succeed at entry if their programs are to be effective. Administrators, who have often come up through the system, may feel that their "beachhead" has already been established by experience or by the authority of their title/position. However, they may face teacher or principal resistance if they try to reenter the local schools.

Principals may benefit from this book. Although they are not consultants themselves, they may find ways of facilitating cooperation with inside and outside consultants, with a goal of building a more effective school program.

Teachers as well are likely to benefit from the material in this volume. As they increase their awareness of the consulting role and its goals, they will be better able to interact with the consultant.

Students, especially those in graduate school in human services fields, including education, psychology, speech, and educational administration, may find this book useful. Many students complain that their classes do not teach them the realities of the schools. Although I do not pretend to deal with such a wide topic, the issues of entry covered here should have real application for students as they finish their coursework and begin careers in school settings.

In an earlier article with a colleague (Marks & Rodwin, 1985), I discussed the individual clinical approach to student and teacher as a means of focusing on the entire class, school, administrators, and curriculum. Such an approach—"holistic or systemic consultation"— views a referral to a special services team or consultant as an opportunity to influence more than one student, and to get the school itself to be more responsive to the needs of teachers and students. A key problem with implementing such a holistic approach is how to *enter* the system at the school building level, and how to convince administrators to permit such a broader function. This book attempts to solve the dilemma, as well as to suggest ways of overcoming the barriers to traditional consultation. The inability to achieve effective entry into schools is often a major barrier to effective consulting.

Although writers have addressed the issue of entry as early as 1967 (Newman), 1970 (Caplan), and more recently (Meyers, Parsons, & Martin, 1979; Sarason, 1982; Conoley & Conoley, 1982; Parsons & Meyers, 1984; Idol & West, 1987; Gutkin & Curtis, 1990; Idol, 1988), issues of entry need to be considered in more detail because they often are ignored in practice.

Writers such as Gutkin and Curtis (1990) and West and Cannon (1988) have suggested facilitating consultation via a genuine collaborative relationship, developing effective communication with the teacher via empathy, paraphrasing, and so on. Their publications, along with the bulk of the literature (see especially Bergan, 1985; Idol,

1983, Idol & West, 1987), deal with consultation on the individual, clinical level; that is, how to help teachers cope with the learning or behavioral problems students face. An increasing number of authors in recent years have emphasized a more systemic or organizational development approach to school consulting (Sarason, 1982; Parsons & Meyers, 1984; Alpert & Silverstein, cited in Bergan, 1985; Zins, Curtis, Graden, & Ponti, 1988; Conoley & Conoley , 1988; Curtis & Meyers, 1985; Schmuck, 1990; Zins, 1992). Of course, Caplan (1970) pioneered such an approach with his administrative consultation.

In the following pages, I try to guide the reader toward more easily obtaining entry to do a traditional consultation and focusing the consultation holistically on the larger system, in order to have an impact on more students as well as on school programs.

This book culls strategies from the work of others in gaining entry and doing a broader kind of consultation, while emphasizing my practical, everyday experiences in the Trenton, New Jersey, schools. Various consulting approaches are also reviewed and defined. The goal is to provide techniques that are immediately useful to practitioners interested in implementing a consultation role and to help otherwise knowledgeable educational, counseling, psychological, and mental health personnel with the nuts and bolts of opening doors so that their consultation skills can be utilized.

Acknowledgments

I wish to acknowledge Professor Joseph Zins, University of Cincinnati, for reviewing parts of the manuscript and for his helpful comments and encouragement. I am also most appreciative of the assistance of Professor George Albee, Department of Psychology at University of Vermont (UVM); Professor Martha Fitzgerald, Department of Special Education at UVM; and Professor Bruce Compas, Department of Psychology at UVM in obtaining reference materials and for their helpful comments and advice.

Professor Irwin Hyman of Temple University's school psychology program helped fuel my interest in this area. And Judi Edwards, School Social Worker in Albany, Oregon, helped critique my work.

The support of Dr. Eugene Gadson, former Director of Special Pupil Services for the Trenton Board of Education, and his Supervisor of Child Study Teams, Dr. Naomi Lennox, made possible the consultation projects that are the basis for this book. The projects could not have been carried out without the efforts of Child Study Team colleagues (the late) Helen Rodwin, Learning Consultant, and Joel Weisenberg, School Social Worker, who helped, encouraged, critiqued, and made convention presentations with me.

The backing of numerous caring administrators and principals made my job a pleasure, as did many of the sensitive vice and assistant principals, teachers, counselors, and staff of the Trenton, New Jersey, public schools.

Professor Leroy Olson, Chair of Temple University's Educational Administration Department, provided encouragement and gave me the final push to write this book. His is a unique approach: teaching graduate students supervisory methods while building in them the key element of self-esteem, which he feels the consultant must have if he/she is to encourage self-esteem in teachers.

I am grateful for the patience, perceptiveness, editing skill, kindness, and professionalism of the editors and staff at The Guilford Press in helping to bring this manuscript to publishable quality, especially the ongoing efforts of my production editor, Anna Brackett.

My son Steven Marks, daughter Mindy Marks-Rose, and her husband, Dr. Mark Rose, helped immensely in producing the figures. My son Howard Marks provided critiques, feedback from staff and graduate students at University of Northern Colorado, and encouragement to keep me on task.

My father, Samuel A. Marks, who died while I was writing this book; my mother, Grace Cannon Marks; uncle Max Barsky, and daughter-in-law Linda Marks continued their encouragement over the years.

My wife, Bobbi, makes all things possible. Her constant encouragement and her ability to remain objective and refine my literary meanderings have been most appreciated.

Contents

PART IV CULMINATION OF EFFECTIVE ENTRY

I

INTRODUCTION

1

An Overview of Critical Issues in School Consultation

This is a "how to" book for consultants who hope to gain entry into schools and do consultation that has a systemic impact. The entry strategies are based on my inner-city child study team experiences in the Trenton, New Jersey, public schools. (See "The Team Consultation Project" section, later in this chapter, for elaboration.) Much of the work involved inner-city minority special and regular education populations. The strategies utilize the philosophies of Tom Jackson (1977) and others, with special attention to the writings of Meyers (Meyers, Parsons, & Martin, 1979; Parsons & Meyers, 1984; Curtis & Meyers, 1985; Meyers, 1989) in revising the consultation model used by Caplan (1970). Jackson's theories deal with the job setting, how to get to do what you want to do, and how to advance by tuning in to the priorities of supervisors.

In this chapter, I offer various definitions of consultation, selectively review some of the major consultation approaches, and look at the stages of consultation (as stages are critical in understanding entry issues). I outline some of the features of the team's use of a holistic approach to facilitating systemic consultation and discuss how these factors relate to Meyers's and Jackson's work. I explore the concept of entry and how major authors have viewed it, and look at the importance of role expansion for special services personnel.

DEFINITIONS

Traditional consultation is designed to solve problems and, in doing so, to spread expertise so that more people can benefit than might from one-on-one consultation with a student. Albee (1984), Sarason (1982), and the Commission on the Prevention of Mental–Emotional Disabilities (1987) have said that there will never be enough specialists to deal with mental health problems and have argued for a more holistic, preventive approach to improving mental health. Their views support the efforts of consultation to change schools at a more systemic level. Although Albee's concentration on primary prevention covers all of society, not just schools, it provides the raison d'être for promoting and expanding consultation. Mental health issues are a key problem in education today and they provide the justification for many of the early consultation efforts by outside consultants such as Caplan (1970) and Sarason, Levine, Goldenberg, Cherlin, and Bennett (1966), as well as more recent consultants such as Zins, Conyne, and Ponti (1988) and Cowen and Hightower (1990).

Consultation has been often defined as a problem-solving process among professionals. A widely used term today is "collaborative consultation" (West & Idol, 1990). The term "collaborative" was used much earlier. For example, Medway (1979) similarly defined consultation as "collaborative problem solving between a . . . consultant and one or more persons (consultees) who are responsible for providing some sort of psychological assistance to another (the client)" (p. 276). Consultation is not a technique but an interpersonal process (Meyers et al., 1979) that has goals of preventing problems in learning and behavior, remediating these problems, and coordinating instructional programs (West & Idol, 1990). Collaborative consultation "is an interactive process which enable[s] people with diverse expertise to generate creative solutions to mutually defined problems. The outcome is enhanced, altered, and different from the original solutions that any team member would produce independently" (Idol, Paolucci-Whitcomb, & Nevin, 1986, p. 1).

West and Idol (1990) see consultation as having a scientific as well as an artful base, which includes knowledge of the teaching–learning process and the management skills necessary to ensure communication and collaboration among the consultation team members.

Caplan's (1970) pioneering approach to school consultation was not so different. He viewed the consulting relationship as two experts (consultant and consultee) working as equals in a coordinate, *non-hierarchical* relationship to help with a problem or program plan (Alpert & Silverstein, cited in Bergan, 1985). The consultant must be nonjudgmental, empathic, and calm and respect the confidentiality of the discussions with the consultee.

Consultation also has been defined more narrowly as providing support to regular education teachers of special needs students

(Knight et al., 1981; Deno, 1985). Knight's group consulted on a statewide basis (Vermont), placing a remedial expert in the regular classroom to facilitate the learning of students with mild special needs. This could be a critical function in light of the regular education initiative's (Hallahan et al., 1988) expanding efforts toward greater inclusion in regular classrooms of students determined eligible for special education services. Consultation can be used to share skills during inservice programs and can help the classroom teacher increase effective functioning (Rosenfield, 1987).

Systemic consultation is referred to as organizational development by Schmuck (1990) and others. Organizational development is consultation that attacks student problems by exploring deficiencies in the interpersonal and group dynamics of the school staff. The system is the target of consultation (Lewin, 1976). Such an approach explores the school norms or shared expectations, structures or routings for interactions, and procedures such as how meetings are run.

EARLY CONSULTATION APPROACHES

Gutkin and Curtis (1982) indentified three major approaches to consultation: problem-solving consultation (based on work by D'Zurilla & Goldfried, 1971), behavioral consultation (based on studies by Bergan, 1977, and Kratochwill, 1978, 1985, among others), and mental health consultation (Caplan, 1970). They revised this view more recently (Gutkin & Curtis, 1990), merging problem-solving with behavioral consultation. They called this merger ecological consultation, noting the strong degree of overlap (see below). Other types of consultation include process consultation (Schein, 1987), organizational development consulting (Schmuck, 1990), and family systems approaches (e.g., Fish & Jain, 1988). We shall first look at some earlier approaches to consultation and then review more recent ones.

An early example of a consultation approach was developed by Tharp and Wetzel (1969) and Tharp (1975). They used a triadic approach in which the consultant, mediator (usually a teacher), and student reciprocally reinforced each other, with the student as the target.

Caplan developed an extensive theory of consultation and practice methodology on which Meyers's approach is based. It consists of four types:

1. Client-centered case consultation
2. Consultee-centered case consultation

3. Consultee-centered administrative consultation
4. Program-centered administrative consultation

Meyers developed similar levels of consultation which I will expand on later (Meyers, 1973; Meyers et al., 1979; Parsons & Meyers, 1984). Briefly, they are:

I. Direct service to the student
II. Indirect service to the student
III. Direct service to the teacher
IV. Service to the system

Caplan's client-centered case consultation is similar to Meyers's Levels I and II, in which the consultant focuses on the problems in the *client*. Consultee-centered case consultation parallels Meyers's Level III, in which the focus is on the *teacher*. Here Caplan dealt with such issues as the teacher's lack of knowledge, skill, self-confidence, and professional objectivity.

Lack of knowledge is often simply a lack of information. In this area, teachers may be made aware of recent research findings, such as the effects of time on task in improving reading proficiency. Lack of skill can be remedied by learing how to reflect student feelings, to record student behavior rates, or to reinforce positive behaviors. Lack of self-confidence is more an issue of the teacher's personality. Teachers lacking in assertive skills may not have the confidence to reach out and move around the room, touching base with each student (instead of safely staying behind the desk). (One teacher I knew would not even encourage classroom discussion because she feared losing control of the students.) Lack of objectivity might refer to such issues as favoring a particular approach to learning even if it has not been effective.

Especially regarding the latter, Caplan (1970) was particularly concerned with clinical issues such as the teacher's overinvolvement, over-identification with the case, transference distortions (being too negative or positive toward a student), overt psychiatric disorders, and/or theme interference (the consultee's unresolved stresses displaced onto the student). Caplan did not feel that the consultant should deal directly with the consultee's mental health, but he did stress awareness of these issues in helping consultees to cope. He would often use parables to reduce the threat to the consultee (note the current emphasis in the psychotherapy literature on story telling and metaphor).

In consultee-centered administrative consultation (which Caplan viewed as being the most demanding on the consultant), the focus is on improving program and management, with the emphasis on staff communication, trust, and utilization of knowledge of the organization's policies.

In program-centered administrative consultation, one of the early systemic approaches, the emphasis is on *program* planning, policy, and organizational problems, with top-level administration as the consultee. These program-oriented types of consultation fall under Meyers's Level IV consultation.

Other early proponents of consultation in the schools included Newman and Sarason. Newman (1967) was also an outside consultant. She saw the consultant role as providing knowledge of mental health, child development, and group dynamics. Sarason et al. (1966), Sarason (1982), and Brown (1985) agreed with her views regarding the importance of changing the school *environment.* Newman, however, stressed the need to accept the school as it is and not change the power structure, as the consultant is a guest there. She saw the consultant achieving change by increasing communication and decreasing teacher isolation. Bringing the staff together in such a way prevents the consultant from receiving a fragmented view of the student. Newman stressed the importance of understanding such group issues as leadership patterns, decision making, and the communications structure.

Newman noted that consultants must establish boundaries between the consultee and themselves and yet be flexible and step out of their role as needed once those boundaries are established. (Caplan, however, was more rigid about role maintenance.) Newman also felt that the consultant needed to be in the school once a week for at least a year in order to gain the confidence of the staff, a concern that remains important today (Zins, 1992). She recognized too that when the larger society lacks readiness for change, such change efforts are resisted. Therefore, the consultant must view individual problems in that larger context.

Sarason (1982) also emphasized an environmental, holistic approach to developing programs. He said that the purpose of consultation was to eliminate the need for the consultant. He saw the relationship between consultant and consultee as a "partnership" and felt that entry was the only stage of consultation. The consultant needs to become part of the school "culture" because a sustained relationship is necessary to develop teachers' roles as applied psychologists, social workers, and educators (Alpert & Silverstein, cited in Bergan, 1985). Sarason (1982) noted that a consultant cannot ignore his/her *own* culture and how that influences the way the consultant judges schools. The consultant must study the research on how schools change, formulate goals for change that take into account the resources available in a school, and be able to muster those resources, in part, by building constituencies and helping teachers "own" the process of change. Sarason said that to change the system, consultants must include targets outside the school, such as courts, politicians, and state agencies. By doing this, he took a broader systemic approach than did Caplan in his program-centered administrative consultation.

Sarason's work, which focused on school *change*, studied the existing regularities in a school, both behavioral and programmatic. He recognized that if change were to take place, these regularities could not be taken for granted. He gave as an example the fact that math classes are taught one period a day, 5 days a week for 12 school years. This assumption is accepted by most schools without question, and much resistance arises if it is challenged. Yet such questioning is often the task of the consultant when attempting entry and subsequent systemic change.

MORE RECENT CONSULTATION APPROACHES

Schmuck (1990) and Alpert and Meyers (1983) were also aware of such programmatic regularities. They claimed that the consultee would become more effective if taught by the consultant to deal with organizations. Usually working as an outside consultant, Schmuck (1990) posited an ecological, organizational development approach to consultation in which, instead of placing on the *student* the responsibility for adapting to the school culture, the counselor instead asks: What are the deficiencies in the interpersonal and group dynamics of the *staff*?

Schmuck, like Sarason, studied the characteristics of the social systems in the schools and evaluated how organizations problem solve, how effectively the subsystems of the organization operate, and how the staff needs for affiliation, achievement, and power are being met. He targeted for change people's interpersonal skills, the norms and roles of the subsystems, and the school's capacity for problem solving.

His consultative methods were group oriented and included games training to bring up unshared feelings, using data for feedback to consultees, group confrontation in which feelings are presented to group members, and process observation and feedback in which the consultant shares impressions about how group members work together. He also recommended a more global approach to consultation called advocacy consultation. Here the consultant tries to change society through organizing to confront the power structure and through the use of negotiation and mediation.

Schmuck (1990) also cited Alpert's approaches to changing consultees via instruction, role modeling, support, encouragement and ventilation of feelings and the use of behavioral observations to establish baselines, gather and analyze data, set objectives, intervene, and finally withdraw and evaluate.

Bergan and Schnaps (cited in Alpert & Meyers, 1983) took a different kind of systemic view and coupled that with microinvestigation of academic learning time (ALT). Here the systemic goal is to improve *institutional* practices in such areas as how much time is spent in the actual learning process. Bergan and Schnaps used verbal coding of the consultation process to be sure it was proceeding appropriately (see also Kratochwill & Bergan, 1990). They were particularly interested in the "elicitors," key words spoken by the consultant to help the consultee become more active in the process. Such microresearch can lead to systemic change if the consultant has a holistic view.

Rosenfield's (1987) work in instructional consultation posited that most behavioral and academic problems can be dealt with *in* the classroom by the teacher, with appropriate modifications to the curriculum and an academic approach to the student. She tried to relieve the burden of referrals to special education by placing key responsibility on the teacher, with help and support from the consultant. She viewed many problems as the result of inappropriate placement of the student in the scope and sequence of the curriculium so that the student is not being dealt with at instructional levels.

STAGES OF CONSULTATION

Understanding the steps or stages through which consultation moves is important to mastering skills of entry.

In Caplan's (1970) work, the consultant was usually from the outside. Caplan felt that in the *initial stage* of consulting, the consultant must obtain sanction in the form of a consultation contract. This is an agreement (though not a legal document) between the consultant and consultee (usually the school superintendent or other official), which emphasizes what issues will be dealt with and what mutual behaviors are expected. Sanction starts at the top and goes down through the various layers of administration (see also Schroeder & Miller, 1981; Sarason, 1982; Curtis & Meyers, 1985). The contract should include how often and for how long the consultant will visit, how the consultant and consultee will communicate, what kinds of cases will be dealt with, whether the consultation will be case or program centered, what kind of help will be offered, and issues of confidentiality. Contracts should also specify what will not be offered (e.g., intervention in staff conflicts and psychotherapy). How each would benefit, including monetarily, should also be discussed. Provision for systematic review and revision should also be written in and the contract must be properly communicated to the various consultees through group meetings. The consultant must take responsibility for this.

In the *second stage*, Caplan recommends that case consultation last one to three sessions, with a focus on the consultee's performance and not on his/her mental health. In this second stage his plan is to (1) collect information, (2) make a plan, and (3) implement it.

Alpert and Silverstein (cited in Bergan, 1985) specified three stages altogether: entry, problem identification, and finally termination (or problem resolution). Alpert and Silverstein's view was also systemic in that the integration of the consultant into the school was critical.

Problem-solving behavioral consultation (PSBC) (Piersal, cited in Bergan, 1985) pulls together elements of problem-solving and behavioral consultation methods that have many similarities. In this type of consultation, the phases of the problem-solving process are first identified:

1. Acquire a problem-solving *set*.
2. Define and clarify the problem operationally.
3. Analyze the ecological situation (the antecedents and consequences of the trageted behavior).
4. Generate alternative strategies.
5. Evaluate the strategies and implement the ones that are chosen.
6. Evaluate the results and start over if necessary.

PSBC can be condensed into stages of (1) problem identification, (2) problem analysis, (3) plan implementation, and (4) plan and problem evaluation.

West and Idol (1990) identified the following stages of consultation, which also resemble those of Lippitt and Lippitt (1986, cited in Zins & Illback, 1993): (1) entry and goal setting, (2) problem identification, (3) intervention recommendations, (4) implementation recommendations, (5) evaluation, and (if necessary) (6) redesign.

These four approaches—Caplan's, Albert and Silverstein's, the PSBC, and West and Idol's—have some similarities, but the most important difference is in the emphasis on entry in all but the PSBC. Brown (1985) also viewed entry, or building the relationship, as the first step in consultation. Brown (1985) developed a similar set of stages but placed goal setting *after* a clear identification of the problem.

Curtis and Meyers (1985) agree that much time must be spent on problem identification, for if good identification occurs, solutions almost invariably follow.

Schmuck's (1990) organizational development stages are (1) start-up and contract building, (2) diagnosing present functioning (includes data gathering), (3) designing the intervention, (4) executing and assessing the design, (5) termination, and (6) institutionalizing. The latter stage refers to the institution's actually establishing new norms and procedures such that continuous problem solving is supported without the presence of the consultant. Many consultation approaches neglect this key factor.

Hence, it becomes apparent that as consulting has progressed over the years, the emphasis on entry and problem identification and analyses has greatly increased. Most authors agree on the following steps in the consultative process:

1. Entry (to include contract building and sanction)
2. Problem definition
3. Problem analysis using data collection
4. Goal setting
5. Implementation
6. Evaluation
7. Institutionalization

TARGETING CONSULTATION

Once we understand the steps to take in consultation, the targets of consultation can be considered. If effective entry is to be achieved, it is important to understand the targets.

An early pioneer in school consulting, Newman (1967) viewed the consultant's initial target as helping an individual student (at the request of a teacher or administrator), then moving toward increasing trust with a teacher to work on the teacher's competence, and eventually discussing professional issues such as theories of education.

Meyers's model resembles this somewhat but he originally viewed the consultation process from four possible levels of intervention. More recently, however (Meyers, 1989), he reduced these to three levels: service to the student, service to the teacher, and service to the system. However, the four-level approach is used in this book, as it was the model at the time my project was active.

Level I consultation focuses on the student and how to provide help on an individual basis. A Level I intervention for Meyers could involve observing or providing counseling to a disruptive student or evaluating academic skill levels. Most traditional assessment approaches occur at Level I and deal with student skills, abilities, and personality; deficits; and remedial needs. However, Parsons and Meyers (1984) propose an assessment model that moves away from traditional normed testing to focus on evaluating behavior as a function of the client, the task, and the environment (p. 125). They suggest three phases:

1. Global assessment (interviews and informal observations)
2. Focused assessment (structured interviews) (see Ysseldyke & Christenson, 1986, and Kratochwill & Bergan, 1990) and formal observations, including a variety of normed and criterion-referenced tests
3. Testing interactive hypotheses, which involve trial intervention approaches

A Level II consultation attempts to service the student indirectly through intervention of the teacher or other school staff. This is both an assessment and intervention mode. There are four types of such assessment (Meyers et al., 1979):

1. Behavioral recordings by the teacher of antecedents, events, and consequences
2. In-class observation of the teacher–child interaction by a paraprofessional
3. Classroom observation of the referred student
4. Observation of other students in the class

Helping a teacher implement an individualized approach to structuring a lesson and showing the teacher how to observe and reinforce a given student's behavior systematically are examples of Level II interventions. The use of other interventions, including empowering the referred student, also expands the impact of consultation. The goal of the interventions is building competence in the student, with focus on growth and development, not just problem remediation (Parsons & Meyers, 1984).

At Level III, the focus is entirely on the teacher or consultee. Here the consultant helps change the consultee, modifying attitudes and providing information the consultee needs to improve teaching; helps teachers cope more effectively with system demands (such as expectations of administrators); or helps the consultee increase skills in some area such as handling students or preventing students from cursing. Much of Rosenfield's (1987) instructional consultation, which helps teachers analyze how they organize for instruction, falls under Level III. Meyers's approach differs from Caplan's client-centered case consultation in that it does not focus on the consultee's *deficits*, such as lack of skill or lack of self-confidence. Parsons and Meyers (1984) eschew the deficit model, preferring to focus on growth in the consultee without limiting the focus to the consultee's problems. They also place less emphasis on Caplan's lack of (consultee) objectivity, because other factors have proven more salient in consultee growth, especially knowledge and skill development.

Level IV consultation is perhaps the most difficult to accomplish because, like Caplan's administrative consultation, it has the system as its target. A Level IV intervention could find a consultant working on a committee to develop curriculum goals and materials more appropriate to instructional matching (Rosenfield, 1987). Another kind of Level IV inervention would include attempts to change school rules or approaches to disciplining students. A Level IV consultation could encourage administrative backing for teacher efforts to share ideas and support each other. Although Newman (1967) sought such backing, Sarason (1982) noted that it is not in the tradition of school culture for such sharing (via case conferencing or team approach) to take place. Such school culture issues are among the many reasons that consultation at this level is difficult.

THE HOLISTIC APPROACH TO CONSULTATION

My holistic approach could utilize any of these levels of intervention. What makes holistic consultation different from much of the writing on systemic consultation (e.g., Schmuck, 1990; Curtis & Meyers, 1985) is my conceptualization of consultation at any of Meyers's levels as leading to a systemic impact. Meyers et al. (1979) and Parsons and Meyers (1984) take a systemic approach in that they claim that the preferred target for intervention is Level IV, the system level. Although it is the fourth of the targeted consultation levels, Meyers asks first whether the *system* can be served, or whether it is the source of the referral problem. Meyers's group suggest moving down to Levels, III, II, and I as each higher level is determined to be inappropriate for consultation (see Figure 1.1.) The holistic approach assumes that, especially for the inside consultant, starting at the system level (IV) will be rather difficult. The focus therefore is on creating change when we consult, even at

Levels I and II, so that teacher, school, or system begins to change (Ellison & Burke, 1987). Although the initial focus of the consultant is on the student and his/her deficits or problems, the goal of holistic consultation is to effect greater systemic change.

This approach differs slightly from that of systemic or organizational development consulting because the latter's purpose is system change and the entry point is at the system level. Consultants who do systemic consultation are often from the outside, brought in by schools to solve certain problems, usually at the level of major program change. My concern is to help the inside consultant (usually special services personnel who provide other services in the school such as counseling, tutoring, and evaluation of children for special education) to expand from an individual focus by conceptualizing each school contact as an opportunity for systemic intervention, hence the term "holistic." Ellison and Burke (1987) support this idea by proposing "interventions" (more limited approaches), rather than attempting major programmatic changes, as a way for school psychologists and counselors to begin to influence the system.

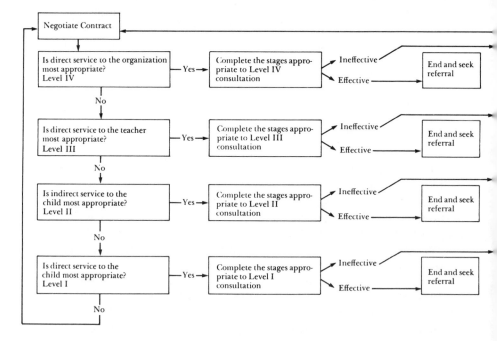

FIGURE 1.1. A flow chart of the stages of consultation. From Meyers, Parsons, and Martin (1979, p. 81). Copyright 1979 by Jossey-Bass, Inc. Reprinted by permission.

I propose, then, that special services personnel work to accomplish the following:

1. Change teacher attitudes, skills, and behavior (Level III), with the idea that changes in these areas can affect many students, even if only one student was the initial focus of the consultation request (Levels I and II). Such change can apply to groups of teachers (Level IV) as well as to individuals.
2. Change school policies and rules (Level IV).
3. Modify curriculum (Level IV).
4. Develop more effective behavior in principals, vice principals, and other educational leaders (Level IV).

In a literature review by Alpert and Yammer (1983), using Caplan's categories, the majority of consultation studies fell under approaches to *individual* cases rather than administrative (systemic) consulting. In addition, the majority of the studies were of a remedial rather than preventive nature. They suggested that preventive programs fall under Caplan's consultee-centered case consultation and consultee-centered administrative consultation. Hence, along with Albee and Joffe (1977), Sarason (1982), and, more recently, Zins et al. (1988), Alpert and Yammer propose that more work is needed with preventive efforts, which reinforces the need for consultants to work at Meyers's Levels II, III, and IV, or for a holistic approach to system impact.

Holistic consultation differs from the medical (or deficit) model by examining the *system* in which the child (and teacher) has to operate. It attempts to utilize and coordinate existing resources to increase school effectiveness. It makes the playing field, especially for the inside consultant or special services team, the entire school and district rather than the individual proclivities of the child. To accomplish holistic goals, I argue for the conceptual integration of Levels I, II, III, and IV while operating at any one of these levels.

For example, when working with a teacher using curriculum-based assessment (CBA) of a student's reading skills (a Levels I and II intervention, because the teacher may participate in CBA), the consultant should look at the teacher's knowledge and skill levels and his/her organizing for instruction and teaching practices, as well as attitudes about teaching reading (all Level III), and consider school and district policies on teaching reading, including emphasis on phonics versus more visual approaches, or the expected pace of the curriculum (Level IV).

Close to my view is that of Davis and Sandoval (1991), who adapted for consultation purposes Minuchin's (1974) analogy of using a microscope to look at families in therapy. Minuchin noted how a microscope used at highest power zooms in on small details but does not see the surrounding field. Davis and Sandoval applied that to consulting when its target is just the child's problem (high-power magnification), the teacher or other consultee (medium magnification), or the broader systems affecting the child, such as family and school (lowest magnification). The holistic approach is like that, though I prefer the video camcorder analogy. We can zoom in on the child at Meyers's Level I, zoom back out a little to look at the teacher and the child at Level II, zoom out further to see the teacher in more depth at Level III, and finally view the broadest field, the system at Level IV, through our camcorder. When we look at a field with a camcorder we see the same picture from a narrower or broader perspective. By zooming out we begin to realize that systemic influences are all part of the same situation, even though consultation may have started with an individual student. The micropicture can affect the macropicture too; hence, the influences go both ways.

Davis and Sandoval (1991) advocate a constant zooming in and out, so that all elements are brought into the consultation and considered together. Their approach differs somewhat from mine in that is uses a structural family therapy model for conceptualizing intervention. They look at boundaries among teacher, student, principal, and others and ask whether they are clear, diffuse, or totally disengaged. They explore the relationship dynamics to see whether the parties are overinvolved, how affiliated they are, and what kinds of coalitions occur (who is allied, and against whom, when there is a problem with a child's behavior).

The Davis and Sandoval model, however, lends itself to intervention with most consulting methods. At high-power magnification (Level I), one could use a psychodynamic, Adlerian, or multimodal (Lazarus, 1981) approach. At Levels II and III (medium power), behavioral, mental health, or collaborative consultation methods might be employed. At Level IV (systemic level), or low magnification, one uses system, ecological analysis, force field analysis, or other means of working with systems and groups.

THE TEAM CONSULTATION PROJECT

Much of this book reflects the experience of a small city's school consultation team, working mostly with an inner-city population, given a 3-year mandate to implement consultative methods (usually of a collaborative type) in order to reduce referrals and evalations for special education placement (Marks & Rodwin, 1985; Marks, Rodwin,

& Weisenberg, 1987; Marks, Rodwin, & Weisenberg, 1988; Lennox, Hyman, & Hughes, 1988). The team consisted of a school psychologist (myself), a school social worker, and a learning disabilities teacher consultant. The students were mostly minority groups (about 80% African American, 15% Hispanic, and the rest Caribbean, African, and white), ranging from middle class to working class and unemployed, with many on welfare. They attended seven elementary and two junior high schools. Since leaving this team, I have added high school experience in the same community.

The team began with a three-stage model in which the special services team member inverviews to define the problem, observes and gathers data, and implements an intervention (Gutkin & Curtis, 1990; Acheson & Gall, 1980; Ponti, 1989). As we worked, we began to develop methods for intervening in a way that could have broader impact. We wanted to affect more students "holistically," following the lead of such authors as Maher, Illback, and Zins (1984) and Curtis and Meyers (1985), Zins and Ponti (1990), Schmuck (1990), and Zins (1992).

When we presented ideas on holistic consultation to convention and professional meeting audiences (most of whom were special services team members), we were met with enthusiasm, and by many questions, which created the impetus for this book.

Some of the questions were:

"How did you get principals to allow you to do this?"
"How did you handle the pressures to evaluate students?"
"What did you do to forestall teacher resentment when you did not test a troublesome student right away?"
"How did you find the *time* to do this consulting?"
"Why would you want to get involved in such complex matters when it is much easier to process the evaluations assigned to the child study teams and keep your job duties simple?"

As such questions illustrate, despite work on school consulting dating back to the 1960s, consulting was far from the norm even in the late 1980s in New Jersey, Pennsylvania, and perhaps many other states (some of these reactions were obtained at national conventions of school psychologists and social workers).

Perhaps we were gluttons for punishment, but we saw a great need to make schools more responsive to students. We also had a more selfish motive: job preservation. If consultants want to keep their jobs, they must make themselves too valuable to be laid off (T. Jackson, 1977). If special services personnel become valuable to the schools in a broader context than counseling or evaluating children, I believe their job security will be increased.

TYPING THE SPECIAL SERVICES TEAM MEMBER

The 1980 Spring Hill Symposium dealt with the future of school psychology, but the conclusions have far-reaching implications for other professions that consult in the schools. One overriding theme was that school psychologists are too often "typed," or viewed narrowly as testers of students or gatekeepers for special education programs (see also Sarason et al., 1966). Though this conclusion was drawn some years ago, the present situation in many schools has changed little. This typing occurs with other special services team members as well. Such typing is aided and abetted by the school structure, with its separate bureaucracies of regular, remedial (Title I), and special education (Ailington & Johnston, 1989). Special services teams are usually part of the special education bureaucracy.

Because of political vagaries, depending on the future of special education funding does not make sense. There is already an expanding movement to reduce or eliminate special education classes (see Hallahan, Kaufman, Wills Lloyd, & McKinney, 1988, about the regular education initiative). Such a movement is necessary so that the needs of all students will be addressed by the schools. However, although consultants could view this as a job threat if they are not prepared for a change in school bureaucracy or in professional roles, perhaps they might instead view it as an *opportunity* to expand their own awareness and consultation role so they can have an impact on all students.

THE IMPORTANCE OF ROLE FLEXIBILITY AND EXPANSION

The Spring Hill speakers urged school psychologists to advocate broader roles, resulting in greater contributions to the schools (which is, after all, the priority, as children and their welfare are the reasons our professions exist in the first place). The consultant needs to focus on a greater preventive role so that the quality of life for students and their surroundings improve (Albee, 1983). This success in developing broader roles, in turn, should encourage schools to keep hiring consultants. Such issues affect *all* professions that serve students in the schools. The implications of Spring Hill for psychologists are also essential to the future of counselors, learning consultants, resource room specialists, school social workers, and other consultants.

What do these broader roles encompass. Essentially, they encompass *doing more consultation* in more areas of the school. Note that the consultation role is not at all new. Sante de Sanctus in 1899 did what was apparently the first team consultation in a special school in Italy (Wallin & Ferguson, 1967). As early as the 1970s, Medway (1982) found over 145 consultation articles in key journals.

But it was Spring Hill that set the tone for school psychologists to assume broader roles and involve themselves more with school administrators, teachers, policy, curriculum, parents, and community. Broader roles involve engaging the *system* instead of viewing the problem as being within the child (Hodges, 1980; Schmuck, 1982, 1990). Broader roles mean looking to prevention, not just remediation. Parsons and Meyers (1984) emphasized the preventive value of consultation, expressing concern that too often a student is evaluated but the information obtained is not used as a basis for consultation. This is the modal case in our district, where child study team evaluations are largely done to meet state mandates and are used mainly to develop individual educational plans (IEPs), which end up in the files. Child study team members and teachers rarely use the information in the classroom. Such concerns were also noted by Magary (1967) and Sarason et al. (1966). More recently, Zins (1992) utilizes evaluation only if it contributes to the consultation process. He views consultation as "the overarching framework to deliver all other psychological services." Assessment must always lead to problem analysis and intervention planning (or to making use of various resources).

Broader roles will thrust special services personnel into functioning as *enablers* (Trachtman, 1981) to help teachers and students interact more effectively, to provide inservices to multiply the effects of the consultant's work (Meyers, 1973; Parsons & Meyers, 1984), to share curriculum ideas from other schools (Wallin & Ferguson, cited in Magary, 1967), and to utilize community resources (Newman, 1967; Bardon & Bennett, 1974). Sarason (1982) saw one role for the consultant as a resource locator and coordinator, as there will never be enough in-school professionals to solve the problems of the schools. These authors also felt that life skills training, orientation and support for new entrants to the high school, and facilitation of natural caregivers were further roles into which special services teams and consultants could expand.

Staff empowerment and competency promotion are consultant roles that can help with primary prevention (Zins et al., 1988). Empowerment involves an advocacy role (Brown, 1988) in which the consultant creates linkages with resources for students, faculty, and community agencies in order to alter the power relationships that exist between them. Brown suggests that consultants take greater risks to change systems so clients and consultees can be better served by enhancing their power to deal with systems. Rappaport (1981) contests the terms "advocacy" and "prevention" as antithetical to his view of empowerment. He states that those who advocate for others unwittingly encourage a top-down relationship with those for whom they are advocating. True empowerment, he says, enhances the possibilities for people to control their *own* lives, with elimination of social policies that assume singular solutions for all people. The role of the professional is to find ways in which people handle their own problems and to encourage the spread of such ideas. Role expansion requires consultants to research the natural support systems that people create to solve their own problems of living and then to encourage broader societal respect.

Some school personnel claim that a broader role for the school services staff is too difficult to pursue. They accept society's narrow definitions of the kind of resource they should be, resisting the gamble to go beyond their role (Sarason, 1982) and content to stay in the less risky position of only working one on one with clients (Brown, 1988).

Others worry about job security or are dissatisfied with the role of tester or student scheduler. Vensel (cited in Meyers, 1980) said that 48% of school psychologists plan to leave their profession because they *feel* they cannot control their roles. More recently, Huebner (1992b) studied burnout among school psychologists and found a high likelihood of leaving the profession, a response significantly correlated with the burnout factor of Emotional Exhaustion on the Maslach Burnout Inventory (Maslach & Jackson, 1986). Huebner (1993) found this to be less true among secondary school psychologists, but still, 29% were either dissatisfied or very dissatisfied. Role control issues often are a cause of burnout. School counselors I have talked to also share this feeling, especially because of scheduling responsibilities. Job security (future employment prospects) was an issue at a recent convention of the New Jersey Association of School Social Workers (NJASSW). They worried whether social work would still be perceived as relevant to school functioning in an era of tightening budgets.

Grimes (1981), Saper (1982), and Tucker (1981) all agreed that there is greater potential for role control through self-definition and *practice*. There are really more options to pursue a broader role than are generally acknowledged (Lambert, 1981; Phillips, 1981). One task, said Saper, is for school services personnel to promote their abilities more adequately. This may mean using reciprocal reinforcement or conflict-resolution techniques to cope more effectively with bureaucracy.

The expansion of roles often requires the approval of supervisors. Saper felt that would-be consultants must educate their supervisors to go beyond their narrow perceptions of the consultant's role and function. Role satisfaction for special services personnel may be greatly increased for those who have the courage to step away from the roles of special education gatekeeper (Ysseldyke, 1984), scheduler, and paper pusher. They must try *proactively*, even in small ways, to improve the educational system (Trachtman, 1981; Grimes, 1981), perhaps by becoming more of a "school engineer," trying to enhance school programming (Reger, 1965, cited in Magary, 1967).

Studies of school psychologists use of time indicate that they spend 7% to 18% of their time consulting with teachers and school staff (Huebner, 1993; Hyman, 1982; LaCayo, Sherwood, & Morris, 1981), while evaluations take up considerably more time: 34% (Hyman, 1982) to 36% (Huebner, 1993). These figures have held up over 11–12 years despite all the literature on the need to increase consulting activities. This may reflect the fact that many school systems reward special services personnel for classifying students as eligible for special education services and punish them for finding alternatives to such classification (Tucker, 1981). Such classification is harmful and also of limited reliability (Ysseldyke, 1984; Gutkin & Tieger, 1979). In New Jersey, administrators recognize child study teams for the numbers of evaluations completed but less often for consultation efforts. In addition, the special services programs in New Jersey are reimbursed according to how many students are classified under special education. There are no funds, other than temporary research grants, to pay for the services of special consultation teams. If fewer children are classified in this way, school funds are cut, with no provision for rewarding teams or regular education staff for their efforts in providing alternatives for students who have special needs.

The separate bureaucracies of special, remedial, and regular education contribute to this problem because they derive their funds from different sources. Yet not all agree that such separateness really helps students. For example, students pulled out for remedial reading instruction often are presented with goals and strategies that conflict with those of the regular class, thereby causing them confusion (Johnston, Ailington, & Afflerbach, 1985). Johnston et al. (1985) note that there is little communication between regular and pullout teachers, so that resolving these conflicts becomes difficult. Supervisors, too, do not believe in or enforce consistency between the two settings, and often the regular education teacher gives up responsibility for the low achiever to the pullout teacher. Such separateness dilutes the effectiveness of remedial (and regular) classes, making it more likely for students to fail and to be referred for testing.

Gutkin and Tieger (1979) suggest that broader roles for special services personnel are possible if categorical labeling is eliminated. They suggest that district special education departments be funded on a lump-sum basis, with *reinforcers* built in for consultees to create successful remedial interventions. The service needs of the individual student should be looked at as a means of determining funding needs. Such changes are beginning to occur in Pennsylvania and New Jersey, where categorical labels are being dropped and services to students emphasize more classroom inclusion, with focus on actual student needs. Supports are offered to mainstream teachers by remedial and special education staff and child study teams (e.g., Ellis & Osowski, 1990).

Role expansion is not without its problems. The consultant who is successful at expanding his/her role may have to deal with increased referrals (Grubb, 1981). Some have suggested that referrals for evaluation decrease after 3–4 years of successful consultation, although requests for *assistance* increase (Ritter, 1978; Ponti, Zins, & Graden, 1988; Zins, 1992). My experiences with these issues are reported later, but we also have found that referrals for special education evaluation decrease, while requests for consultation services increase as role expansion becomes successful.

ENTRY CONSIDERATIONS

How can we make this role expansion happen? Caplan (1970) and Lambert (1981) noted that consultants need to develop "entry strategies" in order to become effectively involved with teachers. This issue of entry provides the focus for this book, because it is hard to have an effective impact on teachers, administrators, and programs (and thereby students) without first being accepted into the school and its social system. Entry is defined as "coming into, joining" (Foreman, 1969) with a school, in the sense of becoming a part of that system (Sarason, 1982). Therefore, entry strategies are methods for being integrated into and accepted by a school. We need entry strategies even if we have been employed by a school for some time. We certainly need them if we are new to a school or an outside consultant.

Strategies for entry include a *self-definition* of functions and role, deciding where to enter the system (Hodges, 1980) and with whom to attempt entry, handling contractual issues (Caplan, 1970), perceiving the needs of others, analyzing how complex the system is, evaluating the resistance to consultant entry, and developing a public relations approach to the promotion of entry and acceptance. In determining with whom to seek entry, and with which power groups to intervene, the special services staff's task is to evaluate who has needs in the school and then to find people with the power to make entry happen. One does not attempt entry to a system without looking at the power structure of that system. Sarason and Newman both viewed entry as requiring the permission of the school principal even if the superintendent has confirmed the contract. This book begins with the principal because of the great importance that position has in facilitating entry to do consultation.

Caplan (1970) recommended that entry be made with the *real authorities* in the system. For Newman, only principals who *wanted* consultation help got it. Even that sanction is not always sufficient for successful entry. Caplan (1970) cautioned that consultants must assess the needs and perceptions of *middle* managers or supervisors (this would include vice and assistant principals and department supervisors) once sanction is obtained from higher circles. Without such feedback, the consultant risks being seen as a tool of management to spy on supervisors or teachers.

Caplan, Sarason, and Newman were pioneers in exploring entry issues. They worked as outside consultants, often establishing initial entry into the schools through university teacher training, research, or mental health consultation programs. Sarason et al. (1966) studied the effects of anxiety on students' school performance. Such work made sense to school staff, who saw this as relevant, not esoteric, research with specific implications for school children and staff. Sarason and Newman met with faculty at low-key sessions, described their consultation model, emphasized the voluntary nature of consultation, and gained the confidence of teachers and permission to visit classrooms. Sarason shared responsibility with teachers for trying new approaches, questioned out loud (as a modeling device), and eased their guilt about not being able to cope with every problem that comes along. He showed great admiration for the difficult circumstances under which teachers function.

Newman expanded her role to meeting with faculty groups and supporting new teachers. She worked to improve the effectiveness of faculty meetings and staff communication in general (Alpert & Silverstein, cited in Bergan, 1985), much like Schmuck did in his (1990) organizational development work.

Entry for Caplan (1970) was difficult because of the perceptions in those days of the roles of psychiatrists as analysts and authority figures. Even today, school psychologists and social workers face similar role perceptions. Caplan worked to change the psychiatrist's role, and in doing so initiated many of the ideas we now refer to as collaborative. However, he found that school staff needed much orientation before they would share their problems and participate in consultation.

To facilitate entry, Caplan obtained information on the school's lines of authority, communication networks, missions, values, goals, and traditions. He noted that entry success depends on the consultant's considering such factors as "salience" (how important goals are to the school) and "feasibility" (how practical is it to carry out the project, and whether financial, personnel, and other resources are available so that the project can work). Issues such as salience cannot be dealt with during the consultation planning process unless there has been good initial diagnosis of school goals and values.

There are stages of entry as well as stages in the actual consultation process. Caplan (1970) found that Stage 1 involves the principal asking the consultant to talk to one teacher about a particularly troublesome student, or to evaluate a student. Stage 2 is when the consultant is permitted to speak to the staff on a topic of interest to the school. By the third stage, the consultant can meet with *groups* of staff or students to consult, treat, or screen. The fourth stage involves permission to focus consultation on individual staff members rather than just on students. Finally, the school may be willing to give more power to the consultant, which could take the form of having an impact on school corriculum development, on program priorities, or on policies. Such a process takes a long time. Caplan (and Sarason, 1982) cautions that often more than a year of building confidence and trust is required before consultation can expand to systemic levels.

Entry requires the examination of *patterns* of referrals, to enable the consultant to diagnose problems typical of those confronting a teacher or school. If the consultant can identify a teacher, for example, who is responsible for many of the referrals to a speical services team, or one who suspends many more students than other teachers do, the consultant has an opportunity for entry. This assumes such problems are of concern to the real powers in the school.

ENTRY AND ORGANIZATIONAL STRUCTURE

Axford (1986) used an ecological approach to facilitate entry. He tried to understand the *social systems* of the organization, noting that understanding organizational pressures and power hierarchies is crucial not only to entry but to team effectiveness. Good entry strategies require analysis that considers the complexity of the coalitions within an organization. The greater the complexity, the more difficult it is to enter the organization.

Organizations resist change (Sarason, 1982; Piersal & Gutkin, 1983). If consultation is attempted to improve student reading skills, for example, the result may include a finding that the school's reading curriculum is lacking. This could be a threat to the administration or to an interest group that may be invested in that curriculum. Therefore, entry strategies must take into account vested interests in the system. Caplan obtained top-level sanctions so that he had permission to cross department lines. In the above reading curriculum example, a consultant may have to deal with the English department, remedial department, special education, and curriculum offices. Top-level sanction is required to bring competitive departments into line, so that the consultant can then deal with them. However, such sanction is *necessary* but *not sufficient* for consultant success, because the consultant must still deal with that competition.

Both Newman and Caplan cautioned about becoming embroiled in a school's power struggles; they said that we must be aware of our own agency's policies so that consultation, even once we achieve entry, does not violate these policies. Should that happen, our own agency or department may sabotage our efforts, despite success. This can happen with inside as well as outside consultants.

Successful entry, then, involves an empathic perception of the needs of administrators. Such empathy for administrators and the need to address *their* concerns provides a *proactive* approach in defining functions within the schools (Grimes, 1981).

Kelly (1986) suggested the use of "public relations" methods to increase the impact of and respect for consultation teams at the building and administrative levels. I have attempted to expand on some of these considerations.

If effective entry and subsequent school improvements are to be achieved, another necessary condition is clear, long-term, central office support (Piersal & Gutkin, 1983). If we are to begin to change the behavior of administrators to facilitate entry and holistic methods of consultation, we need to have regular meetings and other communication with them (Chovan, cited in Meyers, 1973; Singer, Whiton, & Fried, 1970). Such meetings are necessary to obtain feedback on the consultative efforts and, in effect, to renegotiate aspects of the consultation contract (Caplan, 1970).

A LOOK AHEAD

In this book, I explore what happens at such meetings, particularly those with principals, and look at the role of the meeting agenda. Special services personnal need to find ways to adapt the agenda to facilitate entry for more holistic emphases. This can be difficult as building-level meetings tend to focus on disruptive students (Fiersen, 1987) and on production—evaluations, placements, and counseling sessions—rather than on issues such as increasing consulting time or holistically expanding consultation to have a systemic impact.

I have attempted here to define consultation and its purposes and to look at early and more current approaches in terms of theory, stages, or phases. Selected literature has been reviewed and the holistic–systemic emphases has been related to some of the targets of consultation, as specified by Meyers and others. I have described our Trenton consultation team and its mission. The problem of typing special services personnel and placing them in rigid role expectancies has been discussed and related to job relevance, security, and satisfaction. Solutions require role expansion, which can occur if the consultant understands the concept of entry. Entry requires role expansion, and role expansion requires entry skills. The consultant needs to work on them simultaneously.

Throughout the rest of this volume, I argue for special services teams and other school personnel to expand their usual job duties into a greater consultation role. This role is defined as holistic because of its goal of taking individual consulting tasks and affecting more students and staff, thereby helping the school run better and make education more effective. The chapter deal with how to do holistic consultation and the specific role expansions required to make that happen. Basically, I attempt to help the reader with problems of entry at the school building level. I discuss how to build support among key school system staff who are in a position to facilitate initial entry as well as the subsequent pursuit of consultation activity.

This book begins by identifying some of the key people with whom the consultant must cope to achieve entry. These key people include principals, a group I have seen many special teams and consultants neglect or even oppose. Other key people are the special services supervisor and central office, which set priorities for the school teams.

The book also considers support personnel, such as secretaries, aides, maintenance, security, and nursing staff. They are a crucial part of the school environs (and often are gatekeepers themselves). The role of parents in making consultation successful is also explored. Each chapter discusses these individuals' motives and needs and suggests how they can be met.

Resistance to consultation is explored and techniques for overcoming the resistance are delineated. The concept of holistic consultation is woven into each chapter to provide a framework for making consultation happen, and the reader is guided toward expanding traditional consulting from immediate pupil–teacher concerns to a systemic perspective. Suggestions in dealing with school interest groups and the problems they pose help readers to expand their roles. Examples of holistic consulting programs are cited. Communications techniques are discussed, and sometimes the term "guerrilla tactics" is used. This is Tom Jackson's (1977) strategy for work accomplishment and job advancement, adapted to the needs of the consultant and the people who supervise his/her work.

The succeeding chapters take into account the importance of logistical planning, especially the day-to-day steps needed to make consultation work easier. They include time management issues, utilization of school resources and sources of information, and turning obstacles to consultation into assets. Turnkey concepts are discussed, such as helping others to do the consulting work, so that the effect is spread. The importance of evaluating consultation efforts is also examined.

II

KEY PEOPLE
IN AN ENTRY PLAN

2

The Principal

The consultation entry process starts with the principal. In this chapter, I explore situational factors that create problems for consultants in dealing with principals. These situational factors include authority lines prescribed by the district and the attitudes of special services personnel about working with such authorities. To help in understanding principals, possible motives for becoming a principal are examined, along with areas of threat to such school leaders. I will try to create a greater understanding of which needs motivate the kinds of behavior that can pose obstacles to consultation entry. Finally, this chapter explores means of changing principals' behavior to facilitate entry and make consultation possible.

WHY START WITH THE PRINCIPAL?

The principal should be the focus of entry for the consultant. Although the consultant will often find easier access to teachers or other staff than to the principal, in the typical school situation the consultant must deal with the principal. Although the district superintendent or director of special pupil services might have hired the consultant or appears to be the key person to whom the consultant is responsible, the true power in each school is usually the principal. The principal controls the territory where the consultant or special services staff has to work and has much more immediate, day-to-day power over the consultant's functioning. In my experience, the key role of the principal is often ignored by the consultant, and this is a frequent cause of the failure of consultation efforts. As J. H. Jackson (1993) has written: "The opportunity that we have missed is that we have not gone to the higher ground and taken the school principal as the primary client in his or her building" (p. 1).

A consultation project may involve the consultant's working with a department head such as the supervisor of special education or of basic skills development or remediation. If the consultation project's goal is to bring counseling services to the students through a grant from a community agency (perhaps arranged by central administration), it might be easier to attempt entry through the supervisors or counselors who would help to implement the program. In theory, these administrators seem to have the most to gain from such a project, as it would aid their departments directly. Therefore, it may be easier to deal with them than with the principal, for whom the project might have a much lower priority.

The principal may be ignored because the logic of the project just does not seem to include him/her. Yet if the counseling services that are part of the project take place and then run into problems with parental opposition or students acting out, the principal inevitably becomes involved in an unwanted conflict-resolution task. Principals are the ones who permit students to leave class for counseling. They need to approve counselors' use of time. They are legally liable for the consequences of every program, and responsible if a new program results in other school functions being shortchanged (e.g., From whose class does the consultant take a student scheduled for counseling? How much class time will the students in the counseling program miss? What counselor functions are compromised if they participate in the new program?). The principal, because he/she has responsibility for the consequences of any program that goes on in the school, has to be the one who defines the roles of staff in planning and implementation (Sarason, 1982).

Working with a person who is more accessible than the principal has other risks. Such a person may be considered by the principal as a "deviant" (Caplan, 1970) individual whose needs do not reflect the goals of the school (e.g., an extremely liberal staff member who has lobbied for more change than the principal desires). If the consultant ignores the principal's perceptions, he/she may put a roadblock in the way of entry.

It is also tempting to ignore principals because when dealing with them directly, consultants risk having their ideas vetoed. This brings the consultant face to face with the main reason schools are hard to change; namely, *the principal is the enforcer of school regularity*. "Regularity," as it is used by Sarason (1982), refers to the principal's (and also the school staff's) needs to work in a predictable environment. It also refers to school procedures that are accepted without question or challenge. Regularities could refer to periodic testing programs, teaching a given subject one period a day for 5 days a week, or job descriptions (who does what in the school). Chapter 4 deals with this topic further, where entry with school staff is at issue. The consultant will soon discover that these unchallenged regularities are among the greatest roadblocks to change. The principal's power to help change them must be harnessed in the consultation effort. Hence, the key entry point for consultation is the principal's office.

SITUATIONAL FACTORS

Lines of Authority Create Difficulties

In the schools I have observed, even when inside and outside consultants have tried to deal more directly with principals, many have had long-standing difficulties in achieving an ongoing, productive relationship. One problem is that lines of authority often are confused. Depending on the school system, some principals directly hire, fire, and supervise consultants and, in effect, are line supervisors. Other principals relate to consultants in a staff, or parallel, relationship in which they do not have direct authority over the consultant. Even in staff relationships, principals I have known like to have the people who come into their building under their control. This also has to do with the need to maintain a sense of school regularity and predictability.

Some situations involve overlap between line and staff relationships. In the New Jersey school system in which I work, principals have some authority over certain consultants, while the bulk of the authority comes from the special services department. In this system, the principals' portion of the authority is to monitor the working time (of teams based in their building) and handle the distribution of paychecks. Everything else (hiring, most evaluation, and firing) is under the aegis of the consultant's central office. What would seem to be about a 10%:90% supervision ratio (principal vs. central office) is in reality more like a 60%:40% favoring the principal's authority over the consultant, because of the key role of time keeping and salary in people's lives. For example, with this authority, principals can control which meetings consultants attend and sometimes how much time a consultant spends in their building.

One principal resented special services teams attending consultation training meetings at the same time that faculty meetings were beng held. This principal felt a sense of "ownership" over the consultants and needed to control their activities. The team's supervisor felt the same sense of ownership and wanted the team to attend the consultation training sessions. The team members were caught in the middle. When principals in line authority situations do not understand the role of special services teams, or perceive that role as a threat to their authority in the school, it presents a real entry problem.

It is incumbent upon the inside consultant to educate such principals through ongoing dialogue about the role and potential helpfulness of consultants. What is at issue here is the increased difficulty of entry when line authority is imposed on the consultant, or when it is not clear who determines what the special services team is to be doing.

Clarifying lines of authority can be difficult. Sometimes meetings have to be arranged between the various supervisors, or memos and directives have to be sent. It is better to let administrators fight out their differences than for the consultant to worry about the problem daily. The former occurred in the example just described and the supervisor of the special services team prevailed over the principal. However, such "victories" can be shortlived if the team does not have good rapport with the principal. Fortunately, the consultants used their skills to help the principal in a variety of ways, and the tension eased.

Other such conflicts around team functioning and duties often occur. For example, if the consultant's supervisor does not want the inside team to do such tasks as lunch duty or bulletin boards and the principal does, the matter may have to go to a higher authority or be resolved via a union grievance. It is possible to follow both procedures: file a grievance and still follow the principal's order. The consultants can tell the principal that they feel the need to appeal but that they respect the principal's right to see things his/her way and will cooperate and be as positive as possible in the meantime. Our consulting team ran into just such a situation and filed a grievance while continuing to do what the principal required. We won the grievance but also worked hard afterward to meet the principal's needs. We viewed this as a more extreme example of Meyers's direct confrontation technique (Meyers et al., 1979). The result was that the principal developed more respect for us and gave us positive ratings on our evaluation form (see Figure 2.1, discussed later).

Special services team members based in a given school are often required to attend faculty meetings. Many of the topics of these meetings appear irrelevant (how to keep an attendance book, procedures for students to obtain lockers, etc.). The special services team members in our school district often resisted attending such meetings. However, after studying guerrilla tactics (T. Jackson, 1977), our team realized that

CHILD STUDY TEAM RATING FORM FOR ADMINISTRATORS

Please help us evaluate and improve our services to you by filling out and returning this brief questionnaire.

Rate your satisfaction with our:	Very dissatisfied				Very satisfied
I. Consulting with students and teachers					
A. The time it took for the child study team to first respond to initial consultation requests	1	2	3	4	5
B. The usefulness of the consultation meetings with staff	1	2	3	4	5
II. Full evaluations of students					
A. How fast students were evaluated	1	2	3	4	5
B. The ongoing support from, and communication with child study team	1	2	3	4	5
III. Other child study team functions					
A. Quality of inservice training sessions run by the child study team	1	2	3	4	5
B. The child study team's professionalism	1	2	3	4	5
C. The child study team's role in helping to improve communication between administration and staff	1	2	3	4	5
D. The child study team's efforts to impact on school programming	1	2	3	4	5

IV. Next year, I would like the consultation team to:

_____

_____

_____

_____

_____

School: _____

Position or title: _____

Date: _____

FIGURE 2.1. Form for administrator's evaluation of child study team. Permission to reproduce this form is granted to purchasers of *Entry Strategies for School Consultation* for professional use with their clients.

attendance at such sessions could produce important results. Guerrilla tactics are those that help supervisors, administrators, and others reach their goals, and that help them become more effective and recognized while advancing what they want to accomplish.

Attendance at the meetings, instead of representing a forced conformity to authority, was turned into a positive opportunity to learn principals' priorities and to orient staff to the value of consultation.

Let us look at another example of how teams can cope with the authority of the principal. Many principals assign tasks such as lunch or hall duty and the construction of bulletin boards. While it behooves special services personnel to resist the imposition of such duties, which can have the effect of diluting the team's function, good use can be made of such situations. The bulletin board can be a public relations tool to teach staff what the consultants really can do. The consultant can use text or pictures to explain consultation and how it can be beneficial to staff. Consultants can exhibit such tools as classroom observation forms or post research reports on what constitutes good instructional practice. Successful behavior management techniques developed during consultation sessions can be exhibited on bulletin boards.

Lunch or hall duty can be a good way of getting to know students and observing behavioral patterns that differ from those seen in the more structured classroom situations, and may even provide a chance to do some group activity work with students. It can suggest interventions with teachers (based on observations of how they handle students in this less structured setting).

Consultants' Attitudes about Working with Authority

Consultants and/or special services personnel often view principals as a threat to their own professional image. This is especially true when consultants have to work in a line relationship under the principal's authority. Consultants have worked hard for their degrees in such diverse areas as psychology, counseling, social work, and remedial fields and want to be recognized for their professionalism. If they have previously worked in clinical or other noneducational settings, they may resent time clocks and such accompanying oversight functions that appear to relegate them to underlings. Hence, in many situations, the consultant consciously (or unconsciously) rebels, and a breakdown in communication with the principal occurs. I have seen special services staff refuse to meet with principals, and in some cases refuse even to go into their buildings. Consultants need to respect the education and training of principals and remember that the principal too is a professional. This requires an awareness and appreciation of the principal's experience and expertise in fields not shared by the consultant, as well as in overlapping areas (Caplan, 1970; Newman, 1967; Sarason, 1982). The consultant must also remember that having to sign in and out or submit a schedule is an administrative reality that has no bearing on his/her worth or professionalism.

Some consultants, forgetting their role as human services professionals, are unable to separate their own unresolved conflicts with authority from the need to use their skills to help people communicate. J. H. Jackson (1993) stated that sometimes this is a carryover from impressionistic student days, which is a "barrier to forming the deep and sensitive relationship with a principal, who instead is viewed as someone to avoid . . . or to oppose" (p. 5).

In addition, Caplan's (1970) concern with such issues as theme interference, as discussed in Chapter 1, do not apply just to *consultees.* It is unfortunate that some school services people feel their clinical skills are only for use with *clients,* and it never occurs to them to utilize empathic understanding, listening skills, and reflective techniques when they deal with authorities.

To be fair, some consultants have not been trained in such skills. Therefore, some principles of effective listening and communication are briefly overviewed in Appendix A. Effective consultants are aware of their attitudes (and conflicts), including their own theme interference (Caplan, 1970) regarding authority figures, and are prepared to work on them positively when faced with authority demands from a building principal.

PRINCIPALS' MOTIVES

Needs for Authority

Some principals, if they have become acclimated to an authority role, are likely to view even the staff relationship (especially with an inside consultant) as a line relationship and prefer to assert their authority over special services personnel to define consultant roles and functions as well as time allocation to various tasks. At first glance, this would appear to be a narrowly conceived power play. However, principals have an often thankless task of controlling a many-faceted program. They often feel they lack the authority to make an impact on these many facets. Their apparent bid for domination over the consultant actually reflects their need to be aware of and control what is happening in their building and the heavy weight of responsibility they bear.

Other principals are not at all accustomed to the authority role. Perhaps some are new and rather uncomfortable exerting any kind of control over their staff (with whom they were on equal footing only a short time before) (see Figure 2.2). But they too need to feel in control of their job and therefore require information and feedback. Such principals, because of their newness to the job and fears of displeasing their constituencies and the authroities who appointed them, may be even more wary of allowing a consultant free rein to run a project (Sarason, 1982).

The increased frequency of lawsuits has made principals quite fearful about giving up control in their buildings. Principals need to know *when* people are in their building, *who* the people are, *what* they are doing, and *why*. Principals require information on *who* is being seen (whether student or staff member) and whether the function is in line with school goals and priorities. Bureaucratic approaches and power are often used by urban, inner-city principals in order to cope with their "diverse constituency" and with school "turbulence" (Duane, Bridgeland, & Stern, 1986). This need, although expressed excessively by some, is usually quite sound and justified because of the difficulties in controlling such schools. A good consultant, therefore, is attuned to such issues and attempts to work with them. Certainly such concerns can provide an excellent opportunity to increase communication and open the door to consultation with a principal.

Task Orientation

Some principals emphasize a strong task orientation (Ohio State Leadership Studies, cited in Sergiovanni & Elliot, 1975). They do not understand the need of many consultants to work with a *relationship-oriented* leader—one who is receptive to priorities of staff motivation

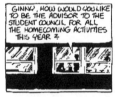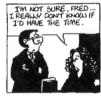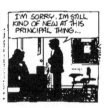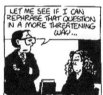

FIGURE 2.2. Funky Winkerbean cartoon. From *The Philadelphia Inquirer* (1991). Copyright 1991 by North America Syndicate, Inc. Reprinted by permission.

and communication, as occurs in Caplan's (1970) consultee-centered administrative consultation. Instead, their task orientation makes them want to see test scores go up, students tested quickly for special services referrals, and so on. They pressure consultants to remove troublesome students from a classroom quickly. Their administrative orientation takes on a "can do" quality of action, an assertive push to get things done (referred to as thrust by Halpin & Croft, 1963). This runs contrary to the orientation of many consultants, especially psychologists, who have been trained to research and examine the alternatives carefully prior to taking action. Many consultants, as child advocates, are not ready to see a quick exclusion from class or a rushed placement into a more restrictive program. Nevertheless, the task-oriented leaders want the problem fixed. Many do not see that there is a connection between staff involvement in decision making, principal outreach and accessibility to staff, and the achievement of production goals as defined by school district demands.

Sarason (1982) suggests that the consultant pay attention to the immediate needs for fixing problems and be willing during the entry stage to forgo for the moment certain broader consultation goals in order to accommodate the principal. This approach is likely to open the door later for the consultant's own priorities. In addition, sometimes a quick evaluation of a student shows the principal that the consultant is efficient and on top of things. If good recommendations come from the consultant's evaluation, there may not be as much pressure to remove the student to a special program. Evaluations themselves can be therapeutic for a student and teacher because of the attention paid and a sense of doing something about the problem. The feeling that things *can* change often leads to actual change.

There are many other problems for which the task-oriented principal does *not* perceive the typical special services team as being of help. These could include, among other things, textbook evaluation, curriculum development, staff evaluation procedures, violence prevention, organizing student assemblies, planning parent–teacher meetings, coping with staff absences, or dealing with visiting evaluators. This is a role perception difficulty, which sometimes the consultant or special services team also shares. In actuality, the consultant may be of great value to the task-oriented principal in areas the principal never thought of.

Ownership of the Project

The principal's needs for authority and control will affect both the outside consultant and the inside consultant who was probably hired by someone else. Yet those consultants often have to work in the principal's "territory." The principal may resent having had no voice in hiring the consultant nor in deciding which goals or research the consultant should pursue. If these issues are not resolved, the consultation may be doomed. The principal's support is often critical to staff acceptance of consultation projects as well (Broughton & Hester, 1993). Outside consultants need to plan their programs in such a way that they have time to put aside their agendas until they give the principal a thorough hearing, and then they should attempt to combine their project with what the principal needs (see Sarason et al., 1966). This may involve a tricky balance among the demands of the outside consulting agency, sources of the grant monies for the project, central administration (who need the money and prestige of the project and who want control over it), and what will realistically work in the principal's bailiwick. It is certain that if the principal does not "own" some of the project, the project is at high-risk for failure. The inside consultant has more time to make this happen, because the other duties such as evaluating students for special education can gradually be adapted to the principal's needs for ownership, eventually expanding the consultative role.

Tom Jackson's (1977) "guerrilla tactics" may be used with supervisors. His idea is that the consultant cannot successfully proceed with an agenda without first recognizing a supervisor's priorities, acknowledging that recognition to the supervisor, and acting on the supervisor's priorities. Although he was referring to job satisfaction and advancement issues, Jackson was keenly aware that such issues cannot be pursued without first being aware of the supervisor's needs. There is a lesson in this for the consultant. The consultant's goals cannot be pursued unless the needs of the person in charge of the territory are consonant with what the consultant is offering. Sarason (1982) points out the tragic failure of many governmental education program grants legislated by experts with the best of intentions. These fell flat because the school culture, which is an expression of staff needs, was ignored. Those cultural issues will be explored in more detail in later chapters, but the lack of participation by principals, who often have the final say in how a program will be carried out and supported, played a key role in the failures.

Consultants should not be so locked into their own role perceptions that they cannot conceive that certain of the principal's goals are relevant to their work. Consultants must not be too busy proving that they are capable of doing consultation or counseling to tune in to a principal's needs to improve discipline in the school. Also, consultants cannot be so concerned with proving that they are professionals, independent of the principal's control, that it hurts to do what is important to a principal. Unfortunately, I have seen exactly this last defensive approach at local staff meetings as well as at meetings on a statewide and national level.

PRINCIPALS' CHARACTERISTICS THAT AFFECT CONSULTATION

Lack of Interpersonal Skills

Sarason (1982) noted that principals, especially newer ones, may not be very skilled in the dynamics of relating to and motivating a teaching staff and, therefore, may see the consultant as a threat to their role and to how staff and administrators perceive them. If a consultant builds rapport with faculty and other staff, an insecure administrator may see it as undermining. Successful consultants help principals to increase their communication skills with their staff (J. H. Jackson, 1993) rather than build their own bridges in competition with the principal's needs. Consultants need to share their knowledge of group dynamics, assertive behavior, positive reinforcement, and other techniques that might help a principal reach teachers.

Excessive Power Needs

Certain people in any field (including school principals), become administrators because of power needs. These people, described by Holland (1966) as Enterprising personalities, value dominance, prestige, and self-importance more than does the average person and are jealous of others who may threaten these values. They enjoy persuading others to follow their point of view (as do many consultants). The outside consultant, by virtue of an implied "expert" role, constitutes such a threat. So does the inside consultant who wants to expand beyond the role the principal perceives as appropriate. Any suggestion a consultant makes could be seen as an implication that the way this principal runs the school is faulty.

The principal sets the tone for the school (J. H. Jackson, 1993). Some principals cope by creating what has been called a closed school climate (Sergiovanni & Starrat, 1988). They follow the narrow view that staff should be seen and not heard. They are comfortable when there are rigid rules carried out to the letter, and they do not welcome change. These principals follow the "bureaucratic" leadership style, generally guaranteed to produce a closed climate (Litwin & Stringer, 1968).

When a consultant enters a school environment, the goal is often to help open up the school climate to ideas and to utilize school staff more effectively. If that does not occur, there is little purpose in consultation. Improving staff effectiveness in coping with students, improving instructional methodology, and other such changes require that staff become open to using their skills productively. Consultation presupposes that the staff is to move in a direction of greater power, flexibility, and creativity, for if they do not, the consultation has failed. As White (1958) noted, people need to understand, control, and be active participants in their environment if they are to strive successfully for competence.

Good consultation moves the "ownership" of problems to the school staff, such that a good consultant works him/herself out of a job. The idea is to create "empowerment" in which staff shares decision making in a supportive environment (Ashton & Webb, 1968). Powerless teachers do not function efficiently (Iannone, 1987); however, they still have the power to undermine school projects if they have not been involved sufficiently in the planning. They may lack the desire to expand their knowledge and skills if they do not see it leading to a sense of ownership in their classrooms. It should be noted, however, that principal power, *if* it exists alongside teacher-perceived power, is not a negative factor for morale and productivity (Tannenbaum & Cooke, 1979).

Hence, the school headed by an authoritarian principal who prevents staff-empowerment can present a special problem to the consultant, because the goals of consultation may run counter to the direction the principal wants.

"Absenteeism"

Still another kind of principal is what I call the absent principal. Blake and Mouton (1964) characterize managerial styles on a two-dimensional grid. The Y axis represents concern for people and it ranges from low (1) to high (9). The X axis reflects concern for production, and this also ranges from low (1) to high (9). A 9–9 principal has a high concern for production and a high concern for staff needs. A 1–1 type would have a low concern for production and a low concern for people as well.

Such a principal (1–1 type) often rules from under his/her desk and is therefore usually unavailable to the staff. Perhaps such people were promoted and took the principal's job for money or prestige but really did not want the position. Such administrators do not want to be presented with problems, and although they may appear to permit the consultant to operate freely, this is often an illusion, a *trap*, and an additional challenge for the consultant.

Like the principal who needs power, but for different reasons, this kind of principal is also afraid to be confronted with challenges and does not want the staff overly stimulated because that would add to the complexity and demands of the job. Such principals are often burned out and cannot deal with the myriad demands placed on a school principal. They fall back on the bureaucratically mandated regularities of school programming and do not want the boat rocked. If the consultant fosters an open climate, with changes in staff assertiveness and creativity or by developing alternative approaches to teaching or discipline (Sarason et al., 1966; Hyman, 1974), the principal may be forced to come out of the cocoon and function. A principal who wants to stay in a cocoon will find ways of subtly sabotaging consultation efforts.

The special services team's or consultant's task is to bring out this principal from under the desk while providing protection from the excessive stimulation of an active, involved staff. One way to do this is through the role of "buffer." Here, for example, the consultant offers protection from the demands, criticisms, and commitments that come naturally from a more open, creative school environment. If teachers want more help than the principal can give in teaching reading or developing language skills in their students, the consultant, utilizing community and university resources, can help the principal set up such a program, making sure the principal receives much of the credit. The consultant can develop parent groups to siphon off any parental hostility toward the principal and help parents act positively to achieve their demands.

FOSTERING SCHOOL CHANGE THROUGH A FOCUS ON PRINCIPALS' NEEDS

Earlier, I noted principals' needs for authority and control. We now look more specifically at the areas that control needs affect, which levels of Meyers's consultation model apply to each concern, and how Meyers's model can be utilized to help the consultant target his/her efforts. Some principals' control needs include:

1. *Controlling the school:*
    a. General building security—Meyers's level IV

    b. Orderly classrooms—Levels II, III, IV

    c. Needing to know what is going on; e.g., in IEP meetings—
       Level II

    d. Orderly hallways, lunchrooms and play areas—Levels II,
       III, IV

    e. Control/improvement of school curriculum—Levels II, III,
       IV

  2. *Controlling the teachers:*

    a. Adequate staffing, as related to attendance and promptness
       of teachers—Levels III, IV

    b. Reduction of union grievances; i.e., teacher complaints—
       Levels III, IV

    c. Not having to deal with too much disciplining of teachers—
       Levels III, IV

    d. Improving staff knowledge and skills—Levels III, IV

Principals' priorities also include the need to meet expectations of their supervisors. Such expectations include:

  3. *Coping with administration:*

    a. Adequate test performance by the school's students—Levels
       I, II, III, IV

    b. Teacher attendance—Levels III, IV

    c. Student attendance to meet state guidelines—Levels II, III,
       IV

    d. Providing adequate curriculum and documenting that—
       Level IV

    e. Reduction of suspensions (often also a district, state, or legal
       mandate)—Levels II, III, IV

    f. Reducing dropouts—Levels I, II, III, IV

Additional priorities could include securing more adequate funding of programs (Level IV), increasing staff (Level IV), controlling parent complaints about the school (Levels III, IV), improving parent support and involvement in school programs (Levels II, III, IV), and creating academic excellence (Levels III, IV).

Each of these priorities, which are control-related, represents a potential target for the consultation effort and, as such, becomes a point of entry for establishing a greater consultation role. We now must ask: Is improving attendance or reducing lunchroom disruption out of the realm of the special services team member trained in reading or counseling? Is reducing staff grievances an issue that a school social worker is unable to address? Here I am arguing for *role expansion* of the inside school consultant, so that target issues such as the above *can* be dealt with in the course of our daily work. Whereas details of role expansion are dealt with in Chapter 9, the crux of the issue is that learning consultants, who were formerly teachers, do know about classroom and hallway discipline (Levels II, III) and do have knowledge of how students learn appropriate behaviors (Levels II, III), and there is no reason why they cannot apply this to other problems. School social workers know about families and the dynamics that govern behavior in a family. Because organizations are often conceived of as being like families (Johnston & Zemitzsch, 1988), the social worker can apply family dynamics or systems theory to solving such issues as teacher grievances and staff attendance (Levels III, IV). However, Merkel and Carpenter (1987) caution that family dynamics do not always work in diagnosing organizations, which have complex coalitions and more sources of power than families.

Arbitrary rules and regulations reflect principals' control needs and can also be the bane of the consultant. Some principals refuse to permit classrooms to be interrupted at all during class time, which means that the consultant cannot enter the class to get a student or to observe and analyze teacher methodology. However, if this rule cannot be changed, the consultant can try other techniques. If the task is a Level II or III consultation, the teacher could tape (audio or video) a specific lesson and review it with the consultant. Teachers could view the tape alone as well if they are sensitive to exposing their technique to an outsider. Teachers can have students record information on teacher techniques or on other students' behavior, and these can be reviewed later.

Often principals will allow students to leave class if it is not an academic class. The consultant may have to send notes in advance to request that a particular student to go to the office. Parental pressure on the principal can also help. If parents really want the consultant to be involved with their child, they can make it happen. Bear in mind, however, that if this pressure undermines the principal's authority, the consultant may win a short-term "battle" but lose the "war." It is better to work within the principal's framework.

Finally, I have been in schools where principals require a schedule of whom the consultant is to see that day. This should not be an obstacle because having such data is a check on the consultant's own accountability.

Another control area is related to individual educational plan (IEP) meetings—those conferences at which program decisions are made about students who may be eligible for special education services or who have been reevaluated to determine if special needs still exist. Many special services personnel resist authoritarian control here and often discourage principals from involvement in the IEP process. Yet the law (Public

Law No. 94-142) specifies that administrators be involved, as they have the responsibility for carrying out the program prescribed by the consultants. My coworkers and I have attempted to encourage principal and vice principal attendance at IEP conferences. Most principals do not really wish to dominate or even constantly be involved in the process, but they do want to know what is going on. In our experience, once included and encouraged to attend, the conscientious principal becomes part of the team and is quite helpful, whereas the principal who is more authoritarian, or an absent leader, finds excuses not to attend but is satisfied that he/she has been invited. Once that occurs, there is no longer an issue about the principal's attendance. In any case, an administrator not attending should be sent minutes of the meeting to keep the communication lines open and should be encouraged to send a representative (vice principal, etc.) to the meeting.

What about the administrator who has excessive needs to be informed of every move the consultant makes? The guerrilla tactic is total compliance. The consultant should send copies of every memo, decision, parent letter, and meeting announcement. Then the principal, faced with information overload, usually begins to discriminate which information is really important and reduces demands to be informed of everything.

This is a better choice for the consultant than resisting the "father figure" by holding meetings in secret or generally trying to exclude principals because the consultant is afraid of their authority. Although this might seem obvious to most readers, I have found it to be a problem in the field with a significant minority of special services teams and outside consultants as well (see also J. H. Jackson, 1993). Instead, encourage, ask, and keep trying to involve principals. The result will be that authority will be delegated to the consultant simply because the consultant complied (though excessively) with the principal's demands. The capable, secure principal will become a key partner with the consultant in accomplishing consultation goals.

Sending notices to administrators and other staff creates other positive results. Consultation is more likely to receive support if people around the school district know about what the consultant does. Sending memos, making announcements, and writing short paragraphs for district and school newsletters all contribute to building administrative support for consultation activities (Kelly, 1986). The school newspaper, often an instrument of which principals are quite proud, should receive regular contributions from special services personnel. Such contributions help support an activity important to the principal and provide an easy route to effective public relations for consultants, as students, parents, and teachers get to know what they do. At one school, the consultant appeared on the students' closed-circuit television morning broadcast to discuss some of the consultation activities of the special services team. They clarified that they did more than just testing and that they worked with all the students and teachers, not just those in special education.

Returning to the principals' priorities, one area of *school control* is classroom assignments (i.e., which grades and classes are located where). This issue is at Level IV of Meyers's (1973) model. In one elementary school, an area originally designed for "open" classrooms was a source of most of the class management difficulties. No specialized teaching related to the open classroom concept was being done, and the area was not physically appropriate to traditional classroom teaching. The choices were to respond to the flood of referrals from teachers in that open space (Levels I, II, and maybe III), become involved in extensive training of teachers in open classroom techniques (Levels III and IV), or change the environment (Level IV). The principal chose the latter, after consultation with the special services team. Teachers who were more structured and able to maintain controls were moved to this open area. The classes under poorer control were moved to traditional classrooms, where their teachers had an easier time managing student behavior.

Regarding the principal's priority of *teacher control,* one important issue lies in reducing the need to discipline teachers. In an urban junior high school, one teacher was criticized by the vice principal because he overreferred students to the discipline office. The special services team became involved in order to evaluate a number of these students. Instead, the consultant suggested a consultation meeting with the teacher to work on classroom management and on his tendency to overrefer. The principal agreed, with the support of the vice principal, both of whom were feeling overloaded with demands from this teacher. The teacher was initially defensive when the consultant met with him, but when it was clarified that the content of the discussions would be confidential, he agreed to work with the consultant.

A program of classroom management techniques; consultant work with the teacher on increasing knowledge, management skills, and coping with his sensitivities; group counseling with the class; and some individual counseling with more difficult students, coupled with a consultant evaluation of the most troublesome one, provided a compromise with which the teacher could work, thus alleviating one of the principal's major concerns. This intervention incorporated Caplan's (1970) concept of creating entry opportunities by working with crises, meaning that entry can be facilitated by focusing on what is immediately troublesome to principals.

Our approach here illustrates the holistic concept in that the special services team began with individual work with students, while having a more systemic goal of broader impact on the school. Level I involved counseling all students and evaluating one; Level II utilized classroom management techniques; Level III involved the consultations with the teacher about his tensions, resentments, and fears of administration disapproval; and Level IV concerned the work with the administration of the school, analyzing referral patterns to the discipline office. As a result, referrals from this teacher to the discipline office decreased, as did the tension between the teacher and administration.

The principal's third control priority is *coping with administration.* An example of this concern is adequate test performance by students, a criterion by which principals are judged by their superiors. A member of our team took on this task at Level IV by analyzing the California Achievement Test (CAT) results of third-grade students and noting that verbal skills were a particular area of weakness. He developed a program (Level IV) whereby students scoring lowest in these verbal areas would receive extra help from a senior citizen tutor (Level II) in building word recognition skills. While some of these low-scoring students were clear candidates for special education referral, this intervention attempt eased the principal's concerns and the pressures from teachers to refer them all. The fact that the project had a clear goal of raising CAT scores as well addressed a key concern of the principal and provided the basis for receiving backing for this rather involved project.

The previous examples address the three primary areas of principals' concerns. Now let us look at some of the means of changing principals' behavior in order to foster the goal of special services teams to open up entry for expanded consulting.

CHANGING THE PRINCIPAL

The Meeting

One place to begin to deal with issues of control and change is at meetings with the principal (Caplan, 1970; Meyers, 1973; Newman, 1967; Sarason, 1982). The purposes of meeting regularly with the principal are usually for the team or consultant to provide an update on their activities and for the principal to share concerns and priorities for the special services team. These include the kinds of counseling being done, which classes and groups of students are being affected, who is being referred to the team, and what progress the team is making on evaluating students or developing IEPs. These meetings are not prereferral intervention committee meetings, although the suggestions below would certainly apply to such meetings as well. The meetings I refer to are essentially administrative meetings to deal with the day-to-day duties and activities of the special services personnel.

Some special services teams do not have regular meetings with principals, while others choose to. I strongly recommend regular meetings. Most principals are willing to meet regularly if they can see a purpose for such meetings. If it becomes apparent that some of their goals will be met and burdens lessened as a result of these meetings, there should be no issue about holding them. Sometimes principals prefer to have the consultant schedule the meeting and take care of the meeting announcements, in order to free up their own time. Meetings should be held regularly but not too frequently: once a month or every other week, so as not to overburden the principal, and to give the special services team or consultant time to produce proposals and results. The outside consultant will also need to schedule regular meetings with the principal, in addition to those with the administrators who brought in the consultant.

Initially, the meetings would just involve the special services personnel working in their typical roles. As the principal becomes more comfortable with such meetings, the holistic consultant's role of improving school communication requires that more staff be involved (to increase "ownership" of school problems). This is true whether the special services team member is an inside consultant or from the outside. Key people to be considered for such meetings, if they are not already on the team, include the school counselor, nurse, and assistant/vice principals (perhaps on a rotating basis, if a larger school has more than one vice principal). The vice principals play a vital role in the day-to-day operation of the school, usually in direct teacher supervision, curricular concerns, and discipline. Others to be invited on an as-needed basis, depending on the agenda, include basic skills (Title I) remedial teachers, physical education staff, attendance staff, custodians, and lead teachers from regular and special education. If the consultant is from the outside, the inside special services personnel/consultants should certainly be invited.

The school should be analyzed to see who the "power brokers and enablers" are (the key teachers or other staff who hold power and get things done), because they will have to be involved in any decision making if projects are to work (see Chapter 4). Sometimes students or student leaders need to attend to present their views. Many projects will not work unless students are involved in the planning. Projects around attendance and discipline issues are examles.

It is not easy for the consultant to convince the principal to involve these people. Some principals like decision making to be their own and do not readily include others. As noted above, the initial meetings might be with the special services team and principal only. Later, focusing on the priorities usually works to expand the membership at the meeting. One principal was glad to have counselors and the discipline-room teacher involved in a meeting when the consultant raised the issue of the high suspension rate (for which the school was being criticized by the state evaluators). The consultant made it clear that by inviting these people, some inroads might be made in the suspension problem.

A school nurse was invited to a principal's meeting when the consultant presented data from a student questionnaire about drug use and suicide attempts in the school. The principal's needs for control of this difficult situation made him receptive to involving people who might have answers. In this case, the consultant learned that the school nurse had a proposal to run student group meetings to deal with the drug issue and so her presence became more important to the meeting's purposes.

The Agenda

The agenda is often the key to making meetings with principals successful. In my experience, principals are usually too busy to make an agenda. They usually know what they want to ask of the consultant or special services team, and that typically involves the progress of troublesome students or those who are failing academically and have been referred to the team. Fiersen (1987), observing meetings of teams with principals using Flanders's observation technique (Amidon & Flanders, 1971), found that most of the time is spent discussing disruptive students, with little left to deal with substantive consultation issues.

To solve this problem, the consultant needs to prepare an agenda to move the meeting in the direction of the team's concerns. I suggest that the agenda be divided into two sections: direct services and consultation services (see Figure 2.3). Direct services refers to the testing or counseling (usually Level I) done by the team and the specific status of identified students. I put this section at the *end* of the agenda once the principal is assured that the team will deal with these issues. This presupposes that the team of special services personnel is efficient and will conscientiously address the principal's concerns with student problems.

The first agenda category, consultation services, includes all the issues with which the consultant wants to deal and, it is hoped, reflects priorities of the principal. These could be such things as improving

Memo To: School principal
From: Child Study Team
Re: Suggested agenda for meeting on 3-15

Agenda

I. *Consultation Services*
   A. Senior citizen reading project
   B. Stress workshop with teachers
   C. Third grade teachers' consultation project
   D. Expanding the resource room to nonclassified students
   E. Workshop for student teachers

II. *Direct Services*
   A. Consultation cases
      1. Referred cases being monitored by the Child Study Team (parent already notified of monitoring)
      2. New consultation cases with no teacher or parent contact yet
   B. Cases assigned to the Child Study Team for full evaluation
      1. Completed
      2. In process
      3. New cases not yet begun

FIGURE 2.3. Example of an agenda for principal's meeting.

teacher effectiveness, dealing with lunchroom discipline, reducing suspensions, increasing students' test scores, and so forth. They are generally issues that deal with the larger school and constitute holistic consultation tactics because they represent systemic expansion from more molecular concerns with the behavior or academic progress of individual students. These tactics are based on the concept that the consultant is more effective if the impact of consultation is on larger units than the individual student (Clayton, 1988). Holistic consultation (Marks & Rodwin, 1985) is aimed at Meyers's (Meyers et al., 1979) consultation Levels III and IV, which attempt to accomplish school improvement by changing school staff and policies.

The consultation services item should also focus on prevention. Albee's work on *primary prevention* (Albee & Joffe, 1977) demonstrated that there will never be enough mental health staff to treat all the problems of individuals, and therefore the societal factors and institutions (including schools) that foster mental and stress problems must themselves be changed (see also Sarason et al., 1966; Sarason, 1982). Prevention can take a variety of forms, many of which could become part of the meeting agenda with principals.

The agenda could include how the team and school could work better with students as a group and with the community. Alpert (1984) advocated changing school–community relationships and the school environment to encourage students to be more adaptive and giving to their community via the "helper" role. Prevention also requires reducing stresses on students, which are inherent in school programs. Special services personnel can work with schools on specific anxiety-provoking stressors such as final examinations (Level IV). Evidence has been presented that at schools that give final exams, there is an increase in student illnesses (Sarason, 1982). Special services personnel can encourage programs (Level IV) that help students with exam-coping skills, work directly with students or teachers (Levels I or II), or even work to change the way students' work is evaluated (Level IV). The general idea is to "empower" students so that they function better. This is done by working with them in changing the home and learning environment and by helping them gain the skills by which they will gain power over their lives and life situations. Such empowerment could occur with a more active student council providing constructive input to administration about improving conditions of learning (Zins et al., 1988).

The structure of classes and how students are placed in them could be another part of the agenda for consultation services. Moses (1991), citing the work of psychologist Robert Slavin at Johns Hopkins, has indicated the importance of preventing stress and poor self-image in disadvantaged students by attempting to "detrack" schools by encouraging cooperative learning (Level IV initially, then Level II and III). Here students of high, medium, and low ability work on teams, helping each other to learn, instead of attending different classes according to their ability or achievement levels.

The agenda could include consulting with staff. Newman (1967) viewed prevention as helping an overburdened staff infantilized by bureaucracy. Unfortunately, her almost 30-year-old concern is still quite relevant today, in my experience. This issue could be ameliorated by Level III inservice training or at Level IV by helping the principal and other administrators examine how teachers can be more empowered and their ideas harnessed. Prevention can take the form of a fostering of teacher partnerships and teamwork (Martha Knight-Fitzgerald, August 1989, personal communication). The meetings with the principal can be the beginning of such preventive consultation.

As the consultant focuses the principal on such holistic issues, the consultation becomes more effective. Many consultants view primary prevention as reducing the incidence of disorders (Caplan, cited by Zins et al., 1988) and thereby referrals for counseling or to special services classes, adding in their own goal of cutting the special education evaluation load. A systemic approach to overall school issues is the best way to reduce such a load (Roth, 1980).

Principals are quite willing to discuss the holistic issues if the issues relate to their priorities. Some of their concerns were dealt with earlier in this chapter. How does the consultant find out about principals' specific priorities? Just ask! Principals (and everybody else) like to talk about what is important to them and what interests them. In many school districts, the principal's job is a lonely one, and principals have no one to talk to about their worries. Sarason (1982) has noted that if principals raise their problems to their superiors, they risk being seen as inadequate in the bureaucracy's value system. If they share with former colleagues (teachers), they could compromise their authority positions. A receptive consultant can be quite appreciated by a principal, whom J. H. Jackson (1993) feels should be taken on as a primary client. Good consultants, when greeting a principal, will attempt to find out how the principal feels, what the principal is doing in the school or district, what today's problems and crises are, and generally what is on the principal's mind. This is in contrast to the consultant typically pushing his/her own agenda. Effective guerrilla tactics require the former if the latter is ever to be accomplished. Good communication will actually create a merger between the two sets of objectives.

Consultants who have not been trained in reflective or other therapeutic communication techniques may want to read Appendix A, which reviews such techniques and provides examples of how to talk with principals and supervisors.

Relieving Responsibility

The successful consultant must find ways to ease the responsibilities of principals. This can be done by suggesting projects that address various problems that principals face. For example, if the consultant has any research expertise, as do many school psychologists and university professors, he/she may be able to help the school write proposals to obtain funding for projects. Many university professors seek out schools as means of increasing their own income (from consulting fees) but neglect the opportunity to further endear themselves to the school by improving the *school's* finances. Knight et al. (1981) used the "carrot" of state funding to get local schools to accept consultation. Research techniques can also be used to identify problem areas. Sarason (1988) noted the importance of data analysis in providing information for administrators to help them make decisions.

Research need not be sophisticated or involve lengthy study. For example, one could examine referral patterns to special services, noting the frequencies of student referrals from certain teachers. Discipline office referral patterns can be studied by counting discipline slips or types of infractions.

Research on discipline slips at one of our schools determined that one teacher was constantly referring students for using abusive language. It was obvious that intervention was needed to help her cope with or reduce such language (Meyers's Level II or III). Effectiveness of such a consultation (which might involve helping the teacher cope with personal frustrations, or with values that greatly differ from those of the students) could be measured by reduction in cursing or in discipline referrals, or even by the teacher's attendance record before and after consultation.

Suspension patterns are also ripe for research, and funding is likely to be available from many agencies, including law enforcement funds (which lately have been more available than other research monies). Suspensions, and the dropouts that tend to follow, often result in an increase in crime; hence, the law enforcement emphasis.

The principal's need for control in the school environment can be dealt with by developing projects that improve administrative control, thereby easing the load on the principal. One principal was observed to be quite harried during daily lunchroom duty. One of the elementary school lunch periods was particularly troublesome and noisy. The lunch aides would scream at the children, only adding to the noise, and the principal was prevented from having a quiet lunch.

A project was developed by the consultants to examine the lunchroom more closely. First a needs assessment meeting was held with the lunch aides to find out about their job perceptions. It was an eye-opener. These aides, all of whom were untrained local homemakers with little formal education, were required to monitor and control the student's behavior, add up cash receipts, check who got government-paid lunches, take attendance, be sure the children ate adequately and cleaned up, and so on, and all of this for relatively low pay. They felt harried themselves, and this feeling was somewhat relieved by the fact that someone was meeting with them to discuss how they felt. They explained which classes were most difficult to handle and had some good ideas as to how to deal with them. On rainy days, when the students could not go outdoors, some classes returned to the classroom to be supervised by their teachers (on their own lunch hours), while other teachers refused this and the lunch aides had to handle the students after they ate as well. Such inconsistencies in staff expectations are a Level IV policy and an enforcement issue best discussed with the principal.

A second meeting was held to teach strategies for behavior management and possible activities that could quiet the lunchroom. The aides were skeptical of some of the behavioral techniques discussed, so it was agreed that the consultant would go into the lunchroom and attempt to model them. The consultant modeled whispering behavior as opposed to shouting and, after observing little or no positive reinforcement coming from the aides, went to the disruptive class's table and patted each quiet student, thanking him/her for good behavior. The consultant noted that 23 of the 30 students were well-behaved. Thus, the description of the whole class as troublesome was not accurate. While this reinforcement of the well-behaved students was occurring, the disruptive students became curious, eventually sat down, and proceeded to talk to the consultant. They obviously needed attention. One began to read from a book and three of his acting-out companions sat down and listened attentively as the consultant and student alternated oral reading.

The result was that the aides were shown alternatives (e.g., reading to the students, whispering instead of shouting, and positively reinforcing the well-behaving students). The aides no longer felt so neglected or left out of the picture. More important, the strategy of attacking this problem gained the confidence and appreciation of the principal (and some wonderment on the part of the assistant principal in charge of discipline). This left both principal and assistant principal more open to other consultation projects. The aides became allies, were willing to locate children for the consultant, identified children who might be in need of attention, and in general were very helpful.

Another control issue came up at a different elementary school where third-grade teachers in a "portable" building had trouble controlling students going to and from lunch in the main building. Here again, the principal and assistant principal were besieged by disorderly students sent to them for discipline. The consultant offered to intervene and developed a program to solve the problem (see Chapter 4 for elaboration).

Consultants will advance on the job if they make the boss's job easier (T. Jackson, 1977). The kinds of projects just described, if successful, certainly make a principal's job easier, and even if *not* successful, they give a clear message that the consultant cares about the principal's needs. Sometimes it does not hurt a consultant to fail, as it then relegates him/her to the human level and may *help* principals and teachers feel more comfortable working with the consultant. The consultant's failure may help them feel: "Now you know what it's like for us!"

In this chapter, I have explored the importance of dealing with principals, the confusion over who has authority over the consultant, principals' motivations and worries, their priorities of improving schools via control of staff and students, and their needs to cope with superiors. I have looked at techniques of changing principals' attitudes and behavior through meetings, the agenda, and easing the responsibilities and burdens of the principal.

3

The Supervisor

Your supervisor's support is very important for entry because without supervisory sanction, the consultant will not really be able to consult. Consultants must achieve "entry" with their own supervisors before they can attempt it with principals or others. Such writers as Piersal and Gutkin (1983), Idol (1988), and Ponti et al. (1988) noted the importance of administrative sanction in order for consultation to take place. Many years earlier, Caplan (1970) emphasized the need for upper-level sanction to consult, but he was concerned with the role of the outside consultant. This chapter emphasizes inside consultants, typically the counselor or special services personnel, and their relationship with their supervisor.

Consultants may have the power to change a supervisor so they can be permitted to do more consulting. Facherty and Turner (1988) indicated that educational psychologists had some success in getting their supervisors to change policies. This chapter discusses some special considerations for dealing with supervisors that differ somewhat from coping with principals. The supervisors considered here include those for special education, special pupil services, counseling and guidance, and remedial programs (Title I), and related administrators.

Much as I did with principals, I look at special services teams' reactions to supervisors and supervisors' motives, the threats and pressures they face, and their needs. I provide examples of how to ease pressures on the supervisor and tune in to the supervisor's concerns through creative consultation efforts and via time scheduling. I explore factors that influence a team's formation, functioning, and effectiveness as the factors relate to easing the supervisor's load.

DO THE CONSULTANT'S REACTIONS
GET IN THE WAY?

Some special services team members react to the supervisor as a
parental figure: They challenge his/her authority and expect love and
support in the form of perks, raises, involvement in program planning, and general praise. They are often quite hurt when they do not
get these (T. Jackson, 1977). They want their supervisor to satisfy
their basic needs for safety, belonging, love, and esteem (Maslow,
1954). Tom Jackson says that such people think they are working for
"the benevolent father" instead of for a fallible human being who may
have inherited the title of supervisor (and who has the same needs
for esteem, etc.). Many supervisors, because of the stresses and
pressures they face, neglect to focus on the needs of employees.
Instead they adopt a style of management emphasizing production,
often abandoning concern for human needs (Blake & Mouton, 1964).
The astute, aspiring consultant will respond not with hurt or anger
but with a therapeutic approach to help the supervisor deal with
stresses, threats, and pressures (T. Jackson, 1977). Many special
services staff members complain loudly over their case loads (and not
always without justification), but again they neglect to use their clinical
skills and listening techniques to step out of their role and see what
is happening to the supervisor so they can react empathically. Heron
and Kimball's (1988) comments on the need for consultants to develop
their interpersonal skills for consultation success apply as well to how
the supervisor is handled—with genuineness, empathy, and in a
nonjudgmental manner, it is hoped. To do this, special services
personnel need to utilize clinical approaches with the supervisor,
coupled with assertive ones as well (see Appendix A). Use of such a
therapeutic approach involves an understanding of effective communication techniques such as attending, responding, personalizing,
initiating, and action (Carkhuff, 1983) (see Appendix A). Carkhuff's
methodology provides a way of organizing the consultant's approach
to communicating with the supervisor. Such techniques assume that
the special services team member has a plan for dealing with the
supervisor and is capable of implementing it in an objective, caring,
empathic way. It is also easier for the consultant to do this if he/she
steps back and looks at the supervisor from a family systems perspective.

Remember, consultants are part of a "family system" when they
work in a school or an administrative office (Shore & Vieland, 1989).
The consultant might unconsciously view a supervisor as a parent

figure if he or she is older or authoritative in manner (J. H. Jackson, 1993), as a child if the consultant is a senior member of the staff, or as a sibling if the consultant and supervisor have degrees and experience in common. Hence, if consultants react to their jobs as if they are in a family, they may develop unrealistic expectations of their supervisors.

In Eric Berne's (1964) transactional analysis, each part of us has a Child, Adult, and Parent which influences our communication. So do all the people with whom we communicate. Thus the possibilities of cross-communication can be complex. Our Child can communicate with another's Child or Parent, and the result will be different in every case. The Child represents the immature, fun-loving, part of us, which is spontaneous and demanding, vulnerable, and easily hurt. The Parent part of us carries the societal strictures of the Superego and chooses to judge others, direct them, chastise, and otherwise do what parents do. The Adult is the more mature part which is able to set aside egotistic concerns and get on with the business of solving problems practically.

If the consultant feels like Berne's rebellious Child when with his/her supervisor and places the supervisor in the Parent role, the consultant risks reacting to assignments and arbitrary orders with resentment and hurt because it is hard for the Child to see the Parent's need sometimes to take tough stands. If the consultant acts parental to his/her supervisor and the supervisor feels more like a Child, the consultant will be giving unwanted advice and getting angry reactions in return. Berne felt that communication goes much better when each participant is aware of which element of personality is dominant at the time, and also of which element appears in the person to whom the participant is speaking. The consultant who hopes to be helpful operates out of the Adult mode but also is characterized by nurturing and authentic expression typifying the Nurturing Parent and Free Child of Berne's typology (Fine, Grantham, & Wright, 1979). Usually the Adult part of us will appeal to the Adult part of our supervisors. This means that if the consultant can maintain a nonthreatened, as well as nonthreatening, stance when communicating, the supervisor is more likely to respond in kind. This is no different from the problem-solving orientation characteristic of the effective consultant (e.g., Idol & West, 1987; Rosenfeld, 1987).

The consultant's awareness of and sensitivity to the family dynamics surrounding his/her supervisor and special services teams eventually may result in many of the perks the consultant seeks. As in any consulting, the ability to help the consultee (the supervisor in this case) think out solutions to problems will help increase the effectiveness of the supervisor as well as make the supervisor more sensitive to the needs of the special services personnel in the school.

SUPERVISORS' MOTIVES

Special education directors, for example, are not out to overwork the consultant, nor is it their intention to neglect the consultant's needs for professional recognition and privileges. However, they all have their own motives for being in their position. Maslow (1954) stated that people are motivated by five basic needs: physiological, safety, belonging-ness and love, esteem and self-actualization. Maslow depicts the needs on a pyramid, with, at the base, physiological needs for air, water, and the like; on the next level up is the need for safety (which includes shelter and protection from physical harm). Higher-level needs cannot be met until the basic needs are satisfied. We cannot worry about seeking love or self-esteem if we do not have enough to eat.

The third level of need, love and belongingness, has particular consequences for the workplace. We are motivated to be a part of a family and to be loved by people: parents, siblings, friends, and the opposite sex. If such needs have not been met at home, we bring them to the job setting. Supervisors have needs for belonging too, and these needs can be satisfied when teams are *inclusive:* that is, when they share their goals and interests with the supervisor. They include the supervisor in their hopes and plans. Many others proceed with projects on their own (see Chapter 2) because it is the easier road to take, as one does not risk immediate disapproval.

Like principals, some supervisors are motivated by power. I believe this motive is related to Maslow's fourth need, esteem. One reason for seeking power is to increase our esteem in the eyes of others, to appear important and influential. If the power supervisors exert comes from *ability,* rather than from their title or position in the hierarchy (Corwin, 1965), it is easier for professionals to accept and therefore to view the person exerting the power with esteem.

However, not all supervisors achieved their position based on ability. Therefore, they need to develop other means by which to consolidate their power. One way supervisors consolidate power is by creating a bureaucratic administration. Unfortunately, such bureaucracies often offer little concern for flexibility or empowerment of the professionals in the system, although, because of their very rigid nature, they help to maintain the supervisor's power. Such management systems often cause conflict with professionals, who would like things to be more flexible so they can use their skills. Bureaucratic systems actually make it harder for special services personnel to hold their supervisors in any esteem.

Some supervisors have sincere goals of doing good things for children as well as for their staff. These motives could come from a middle level of Maslow's needs (to be loved), or from the fifth and highest level, self-actualization. Self-actualization needs seek to utilize our abilities more effectively: "What a person *can* be, he *must* be" (Maslow, 1954, p. 46). Such supervisors are rare and are to be valued greatly. They may excel in their abilities at leadership, inspiration of others, and organization.

Other supervisors may also have strong needs for structure and organization, while some prefer to be task oriented without attending to staff needs. Some are motivated by avoidance and become absentee supervisors who attend to neither staff nor production (Blake & Mouton, 1964). On the managerial grid, Blake and Mouton graphed supervisors from low (1) to high (9) on two dimensions: (1) attending to staff needs and (2) production emphasis. The task-oriented supervisor who ignores staff needs might score an 8 on production emphasis while only a 1 on staff needs. This would be referred to as an 8–1 supervisor. The absentee supervisor scores low on both concern for production and concern for staff and so might rate a 1–1. These two supervisors may have regressed to lower levels on Maslow's scheme, perhaps even to that of the safety level. They may be looking out for their own success just by holding things together in a survival mode.

Some administrators arrived via promotion, thinking that the job was an advancement (esteem motive) when, in reality, they were better at teaching, counseling, social case work, and the like than at administrative skills. They may have been subject to security (safety) needs (Maslow, 1954) and allowed themselves to move up because they perceived that they would find greater job stability, or by achievement (esteem) needs (to advance for prestige or accomplishment). As in the Peter Principle (Peter & Hull, 1984), they were advanced to their "level of incompetence." They might have achieved a degree of self-actualization by forgoing promotion and staying instead with the specialty in which they were really talented. Such supervisors can be reached through tapping into their knowledge of teaching or counseling, reviving skills of which they have pleasant memories. I once had a supervisor who was a skilled special education teacher. He became a director of a special education facility. Although he did have talent for such work, he would really shine when asked to help the consultant with a class that was having behavioral problems, or that needed help in overcoming remedial reading difficulties.

How many of us plan our day with these factors in mind? I would guess that most special services staff do not spend much time thinking about which needs motivate their supervisors. For the supervisor who is concerned with structure and organization, do we make attempts to meet those needs? What could a consultant do with a supervisor with such motives? Simply, the consultant could develop programming to improve how things are organized so the supervisor will feel more in control. The consultant could volunteer to head a committee to develop a staff procedures manual or to reorganize the forms the department uses. "But this isn't part of my job description," the consultant may argue. It is, if the consultant wants to be freer to do consultation. In this specific example, the procedures and forms the committee recommends could help to facilitate consultation. Our team developed a variation on the special education referral form (see Figure 3.1) in which we listed various services and options (in the middle third of the form) available in the school as alternatives to referring students for special education. The top of the form leaves room to write what happened at the consultation conference after a student was referred to the Child Study Team (CST) for intervention. On the bottom third The Child Study Team member reports what was described at this prereferral conference: whether or not the student will receive a full evaluation by all members of the CST; a partial evaluation, perhaps by only one team member; or a referral for consultation efforts, to be carried out prior to any evaluation.

Our willingness to deal with forms helped empower us to change procedure to foster consultation goals. The supervisors' motives for organized approaches and their needs to reduce special education classifications were partially met by this procedural change. It is the consultant's choice: Meet the supervisor's needs and have more latitude to be yourself, or neglect the supervisor's needs, and fail because the supervisor is not connecting with your needs.

One way to meet a supervisor's needs for security is to propose methods of consultation that increase accountability. If a program of consulting with special education teachers provides documentation of student *progress,* the supervisor's needs for control (and for relief from higher administrators' pressures for such documentation) will be met. Many administrators doubt that special education placements work (with some support from the literature) (see Keogh, cited in the regular education initiative [Hallahan et al., 1988, pp. 19–28]) and will look for ways to decrease funds for that department. If the consultant can prove that students do progress, the supervisor's position becomes more secure. The Consultation Progress Report (Figure 3.2) is one means of providing such documentation, because

CHILD STUDY TEAM CONSULTATION REPORT

Date	Consultation activities (record teacher and other staff conferences, parent contacts, phone calls, etc.)	Initials

Date	Report of pre-referral conference plan	In attendance
	1. Enroll in after-school program	
	2. Place in basic skills program: Math - Reading	
	3. Switch classes	
	4. Bring in grandparent volunteer as tutor or role model	
	5. Guidance counselor to provide counseling	
	6. Peer tutoring	
	7. Administrative transfer to another school	
	8. Grade level meetings of all student's teachers	
	9. Screening - specify type : (Vision, hearing, intelligence, reading, etc.)	
	10.Other: Pupil assistance committees	

Circle appropriate intervention:

Full CST evaluation

Partial CST evaluation

No CST evaluation

CST consultation only

Psychologist _____   Learning Consultant_____

Social Worker_____   Speech Correctionist_____

Case Manager_____

FIGURE 3.1. Alternatives to special education classification. Permission to reproduce this form is granted to purchasers of *Entry Strategies for School Consultation* for professional use with their clients.

CONSULTATION PROGRESS REPORT

	Date	Time Started	Time Finished	Total Hours
Consultee: _____	____	_____	_____	_____
Position: _____	____	_____	_____	_____
Class/Position: _____	____	_____	_____	_____
Consultant: _____	____	_____	_____	_____

1. *Identification of problem:*

2. *Gathering data:*

Type	Person responsible	Due date

3. *Setting goals:*

4. *Selecting intervention strategies:*

Level*	Strategy

5. *Evaluation of intervention:*

Evaluation measures	Person responsible	Due date

6. *Conclusion:*
   _____ Intervention effective   _____ Intervention ineffective
   _____ Terminate services   _____ Set new goals
   _____ Refer for complete evaluation

7. *Comments:*

_____   _____
Consultee signature   Team member signature

*Level
   I —Direct service to student
   II —Indirect service to student through consultee
   III —Direct service to consultee
   IV —Service to organization

FIGURE 3.2. Consultation Progress Report. Permission to reproduce this form is granted to purchasers of *Entry Strategies for School Consultation* for professional use with their clients.

the form specifies the method of measuring progress and outlines the degree of success. Finally, at times the consultant just must *do* consultation to prove that it is a worthwhile activity.

Now let us look at some other factors to be aware of in dealing effectively with the supervisor.

SUPERVISORS' PRESSURES AND FEARS

Consultants need to sensitize themselves to supervisors' pressures and worries. Axford (1986) emphasized the need for consultants to develop a greater understanding of organizational pressures. I would add the need to understand threats to supervisors. One way to accomplish this is to use Tom Jackson's (1977) guerrilla tactics. As noted in Chapter 2, guerrilla tactics help the supervisor succeed so that the employee—in this case, the special services team member—can be appreciated, achieve entry, be freer to advance, and have room to do a creative job, including consultation. Consultation skills are often helpful in this task itself. I would like to share my experiences of some of these pressures and needs because I have seen special services team members go on with their work seemingly unaware of what their supervisor is going through. Then they wonder why the supervisor is not attuned to their needs to do more creative work, such as consulting.

Special education supervisors face unique pressures. These pressures include meeting state requirements for reevaluating special education students; documenting their progress in special education programs; providing a "least restrictive environment," as required by Public Law 94-142; coping with parents' demands for the right setting for their child; and keeping to the legal requirements for documentation (regarding how soon consultations, evaluations, and classification/IEP meetings are held; proper notification of parents; what goes in which files; etc.).

Directors are affected by political pressures. Principals persuade them to provide services (having more counselors or special services teams in their building more often), and board members or administrators always have special requests, often because a parent has applied pressure to get services for a child ("test *my* child first").

Supervisors may fear being fired for not meeting state and district demands, may have a budget that is overwhelmed by excessive referrals of students, testing, and other staffing demands (such as the need to create new classes or send handicapped students out of district to private or county/state schools). Special education teams and counselors, as well as supervisors, also feel such pressures and fears, but the implications are most weighty for supervisors. They bear the financial and programmatic responsibilities, which must be justified to their superiors, the school board, state evaluators, and even legal advocates.

These pressures and fears often are displaced downward onto special services workers and are experienced as pressures to evaluate more students, do more reevaluations, determine special education eligibility more quickly, and also mainstream or remove from special education services as many students as possible. The typical team member tries to comply, and in the everyday hectic schedule that follows, little consultation takes place (Johnson, Pugach, & Hammitte, 1988).

Some special education supervisors, under pressure to get more evaluations done, attempt to dictate test batteries to the school psychologist (Bowser, 1994), holding out the carrot of being able to do more consultation if the abbreviated battery is used. In other words, the pressures on supervisors to produce results can cause them to encourage ethical violations. I have seen reevaluations of special education students done by some districts that amounted to a brief observation and a report of one or two paragraphs. Such information would be of little value to teachers for providing proper programming for their special education students. I believe such lowering of quality often occurs in response to the supervisor's anticipation of not completing huge backlogs of reevaluations and the subsequent fears of retribution from higher-level administrators.

The guidance director or principal usually supervises counselors. In some districts, the guidance director is under even greater pressure than the special education department because guidance administrative services do not have the strength of legal mandate that special education services have. Many schools have eliminated the guidance director's job and reduced counseling services as well, to save money in a time of tight budgets and decreasing federal aid. Hence, the guidance director may realistically be in fear of losing his/her job, which often translates into inordinate demands on counselors for documentable results.

Counselors as well often end up with a heavily scheduled individual and group counseling load. Many counselors also have administrative tasks, such as scheduling students for classes, recording grades, sending out transcripts to schools and colleges, and reacting to demands from the discipline office to cope with students' behavior. They have endless paper work, often to justify the use of their time.

Particularly in cities, both large and small, where poverty, crime, drugs, unemployment, and a mobile multiethnic population are present, there are pressures on the special education director to include more students under special education so they can receive more intense remedial services than can be provided through Title I or bilingual approaches. Few bilingual or ESL (English as a Second Language) classes are geared with special education or remedial goals in mind. The increasing numbers of nonreading students from Africa, Southeast Asia, the Caribbean, Mexico, Central America, and South America create pressures not only on bilingual programs, but also on special education. There is also a shortage of teachers, special services teams, and counselors who are bilingually trained. Professionals trained in bilingual skills come at a high cost, and districts, even under legal mandates to provide services, often lack the financial resources to recruit adequately.

The special services team member or consultant must do an analysis of these pressures as well as the needs of the special education or other director and find ways for consultation methods to ease these burdens. By using his/her clinical and consulting skills, the consultant can work with the supervisor and thereby expand the consultant role.

EASING PRESSURES ON THE SUPERVISOR

There are at least two ways to react to supervisors' pressures. One is to converse therapeutically with the supervisor. The other is to help develop programs that will remove stressors.

The following examples illustrate how the consultant can provide a service, achieve an important step toward entry, and, while doing so, ease pressure on a supervisor.

The vocational school director of one district complained to the special education director that students were being "dumped" on him. He was reluctant to continue admitting special education students. The special services team, with the school counselor, worked out a program of vocational screening, including aptitude and interest testing of special education students. We used tests that minimized the reading factor, so accurate measures could be obtained even from the many students who were poor readers. This project expanded the role of both the counselor and the special services team. The students were helped by identifying those with good vocational aptitudes, by giving them an opportunity to explore their interests, and by forcing them to consider the discrepancies between what they said they wanted to study in a vocational program and what their actual interests and aptitudes were. Equally important, the project eased the pressure on the special education director. The vocational–technical director was pleased that students had supporting documentation justifying their referral, and he became more receptive to working with special education students.

Another consulting approach to easing pressures on supervisors occurred in a junior high school where the state had pressured the special education director to mainstream more students. The special services team met with the teachers, developed criteria for mainstreaming, based in part on studies of the educational levels of the students who were not receiving special education services (which were not always higher than the special education students' levels), and then met with the principal and mainstream teachers who were to be consultation targets. Class schedules were obtained so that at least partial mainstreaming could occur, and the special services teams followed the progress of each student.

An inservice program was developed to inform teachers of the requirements of Public Law 94-142, to reassure them, and to deal with their concerns. Although such plans and programs are no doubt widespread (Hallahan et al., 1988), the issue here is the relief of pressure on the supervisor in order to accomplish further opportunities for consultation. This project was initiated by the special services *team* (in response to the awareness of the pressure the supervisor was feeling) and not by the supervisor.

When this project worked, the supervisor (and principal) became more receptive to the team's desire to expand consultation. This included a Level IV intervention (Parsons & Meyers, 1984) to create a schoolwide conference on issues of concern to students: drugs, stress, alcoholism, dating, and so forth. Outside experts were brought in as panelists, and the consultation project also targeted Level II by involving the counselors and nurse in the conference. This further success at entry and subsequent role expansion occurred only because the supervisor's needs were met first.

The consultant can help ease the supervisor's fears of being overwhelmed by bilingual referral demands. When we began to receive too many referrals of English-speaking Jamaican and Liberian students who were failing academically, the special services team lobbied the bilingual department to consider the students under the latter's jurisdiction. The rationale was that the language patterns in Jamaica and Liberia were so different they could not understand the "Trenton, New Jersey" English of their teachers and vice versa. Through assertive pressure, the team was able to accomplish this goal and thereby reduce another stressful issue for the supervisor. The bilingual department agreed to provide ESL services before referring these students to special education.

If supervisors' worries are connected to the volume of required reevaluations of special education students, special services personnel could utilize Shapiro's curriculum-based assessment "probes" as part of the testing (Rosenfield & Shapiro, 1989; Shapiro & Derr, 1990). These probes document the in-class progress of a student much better than do standardized tests, and they open the way to a positive consulting relationship with the teacher because the measures utilize the actual material from the classroom. I consult with special education teachers, observe, and gather data on student progress useful in the reevaluation process. This saves time when reevaluation reports are written.

The counselor who wants to do more consulting will need to find means of helping his/her supervisor justify the need for school counselors. This may be accomplished by creating a constituency (Sarason, 1988) that, by its existence, forces upper administration to maintain the counseling department as a key part of the budget. Counselors can do this by making themselves valuable to other departments through their services, thereby easing pressures on other departments and gaining their backing. For example, with regard to the bilingual problems, why not develop a group counseling program to help bilingual students adapt to the school and new environment? Dropout prevention programs including group meetings and job training encourage the backing of the discipline department and also may enlist the interest of the local media, which, in turn, could reflect well on the supervisor and solidify his/her position.

SAVING THE SUPERVISOR WHILE BECOMING CREATIVE

Tom Jackson's approach is to save the supervisor's position. But, how? Can the consultant accomplish this by getting the supervisor to let him/her do more consultation? The answer is yes.

Good consultation of a holistic nature should reduce referrals (Ritter, 1978), whether to counselors or to other special services team members. It should also lower the number of students determined eligible for special education services (Lloyd, cited in Hallahan et al. 1988; Lennox, Marks, Rodwin, Hughes, & Kaplan, 1986). Working with one teacher may affect 30 students in an elementary school and 200 in a junior high or high school—a task that is much easier than finding the time to evaluate or counsel those 230 students. Consultation that improves a school's discipline policies may greatly reduce suspensions as well as referrals for counseling or special education. Changing a school's approach to handling remedial and behavioral problems may reduce evaluations and special class placements, all of which reduces pressure on the supervisor. Counselors and special services teams should be aware of research that demonstrates such a viewpoint, for example, Idol's (1988) discussion of the costs and benefits of doing collaborative consultation. If special services personnel have concrete knowledge to present to the supervisor about certain problems that could be solved via consultation, the supervisor will want to listen. Persistence is important.

Saper (1982) suggested bargaining with supervisors before fighting or giving up. The consultant needs to be assertive yet flexible with supervisors. Flexibility is required because the consultant will not always be able to do everything he/she desires. However, an assertive stance should be taken to have the supervisor delineate a clear consultation role for the consultant. Haight (1984) cautioned that supervisors must clearly define the role of the special services team, or the consultant risks facing an untenable situation. That is, is the special services person a tester, a gatekeeper for special education, a counselor, or a consultant? However, this ambiguity also presents an opportunity for *self-definition* of the role, though the sanction of the supervisor will make carrying out the consultation role easier. Supervisors, Haight said, need to be made aware of the multiple responsibilities consulting involves and of the need for more professional preparation for staff who want to consult (see also Kratochwill & Van Someren, 1985).

FINDING TIME TO CONSULT

Of course, if the supervisor does more clearly define the consultant's role (to the consultant, to principals, and to school administrators) as including consultation, and agrees to have the consultant do more consultation, the consultant has another problem: How does he/she find time to do this extra consulting? Most educational personnel work a 30- to 40-hr week. If, for example, a consultant decides to conduct the typical course of collaborative consultation with a teacher, using the stages discussed in Chapter 1, he/she would have to start with one class period to meet with the teacher. The two would specify the problem, define it in behavioral terms, and then mutually decide which data should be gathered to help determine the intervention. A second class period would be devoted to gathering those data, usually through a classroom observation. A third period would be used to go over the results. Possibly they would need a fourth period to evaluate the intervention, a fifth to carry out a revision, and a sixth to evaluate that revision.

If these were compressed into two periods a week, considering training in the method and some evaluation time, the special services personnel would be spending 2 to 3 hours a week for only 2 or 3 weeks and sould have an impact on the behavior of 30 to 200 students. This time commitment represents 5–7% of the consultant's time and therefore should be easily acceptable to supervisors. Similar time commitments for meeting with principals or planning programs could raise total consulting time to little more than 10% of the consultant's week, still a small proportion. (See Chapter 8 for more on time management.)

Certainly, it is worth the effort to convince the supervisor to allow more consultation time. One could cite costs versus benefits, as well as the value of doing consultation before pulling students out of regular classes and referring them to special education (Knight et al., 1981; Idol, 1988). In our district, supervisors encouraged a consultation effort by assigning certain teams to an almost exclusive consulting role, relieving them from reevaluation and special education class monitoring duties (Marks et al., 1988; Lennox et al., 1988; Marks et al., 1987; Marks & Rodwin, 1985). If the consultant can arrange such a realignment of duties, time management becomes less of a concern. However, documentation of what the consultant accomplishes becomes even more important, because consultation activities cannot be counted as easily as the number of evaluations the consultant does. For this purpose, I have included the Consultation Progress Report (Figure 3.2). This form, used in the Trenton, New Jersey, schools was developed by our supervisor at that time, Naomi Lennox (Lennox et al., 1988). It documents consultation activities and keeps both consultant and consultee on track. It specifies the problem, what data will be gathered, *who* will gather it, and *when*. Interventions are then recorded according to Meyers's levels of targeting. Results and evaluation are also recorded, consultation is concluded and recycled, or the methods reconsidered. Because both teacher (consultee) and consultant sign the form, there is a mutual commitment and agreement as to what happened.

TEAM FUNCTIONING AND THE SUPERVISOR

Another area of concern for special services and guidance supervisors is effective team functioning. Supervisors want to minimize squabbles and have teams work effectively with parents, schools, and students, and they would rather not be bothered by personnel hassles. The guerrilla tactics here are to foster consultation by *improving team functioning* so that the supervisor is relieved of this kind of management pressure. But isn't that the job of the supervisor, one might ask? No.

As a mature professional, the consultant is responsible for smooth team functioning. To this end, the consultant should be familiar with the research on effective teamwork. Some good work in the field has been done by Ysseldyke (1984); Maher and Illback (1985); Maher and Bennett (1984), using the work of Tuckman (1965); Hamway and Elias (1988), using a form from the Council for Exceptional Children (CEC); Stokes (1982); Corso and Murphy (1988); Huebner and Hahn (1990); and Sundstrom, DeMeuse, and Futrell (1990). It is important for consultants to be aware of how their own team is functioning and how they can make it more effective. A good first step in improving the team is for consultants to assess where the team is in terms of stages of team development.

Stages of Team Development

Hamway and Elias (1988), working with intervention assistance teams in New Jersey (see Chapter 8), utilized NASP (National Association of School Psychologists) and CEC materials (Stokes, 1982) to identify the skills required for such teams (Figure 3.3) and the stages of team development (Figure 3.4). These stages included orientation, dissatisfaction, resolution, production, and termination. Maher and Bennett (1984) applied Tuckman's (1965) somewhat more vivid descriptions of similar stages of development to child study teams: forming, storming, norming, performing, and adjourning. Here the two sets of stages will be considered together.

In the forming or orientation stage, the team members are positive, hopeful, feel each other out cautiously, and experience a certain honeymoon effect in which they are anxious to improve their skills and make a contribution. They attack problems in a positive manner.

In the storming or dissatisfaction stage, the team becomes frustrated as problems arise that are not easily solved. Disputes arise over leadership and influence, and the goals and motives of other team members are questioned. Team members begin to doubt their competence and that of their team members. Tasks need to be redefined so that they are more achievable.

The norming or resolution stage involves clearer task definitions

	Yes	No	N/A
1. Do members have knowledge of informal assessment techniques?			
2. Do members have knowledge of the scope and sequence of academic content areas?			
3. Do members have observational skills?			
4. Do members understand the district philosophy?			
5. Do members have knowledge of the various program goals?			
6. Do members have knowledge of various instructional strategies?			
7. Do members have knowledge of behavior change strategies?			
8. Do members have knowledge of available resources in the building, district, or region?			
9. Do members have knowledge of eligibility criteria for placement in special education programs?			
10. Do members have good listening skills?			
11. Do members have good conflict resolution skills?			
12. Do members have collaborative decision-making skills?			
13. Do members have knowledge of group dynamics?			
14. Do members have sending and receiving communication skills?			
15. Does chairperson have leadership skills.			
16. Does chairperson have management skills?			

FIGURE 3.3. Checklist of skills needed by intervention assistance team members. From Stokes (1982, p. 10) Copyright 1982 by The Council for Exceptional Children. Reprinted by permission.

and production goals. Here the frustration begins to ease as members become clearer on what each is expected to do. Satisfaction, skills, and self-esteem begin to grow.

By the performing or production stage, a more realistic eagerness to be part of the team returns. Leadership, ideas, and values are shared, and people feel autonomous yet interdependent with other team members. Members become more creative and freer to go beyond the usual job definitions to reach a higher plane of efficiency and accomplishment. This is when the team is most effective.

The final step, adjourning or termination, describes what happens when team members complete their terms and leave. There is a shared sense of both sadness and accomplishment.

Consultants can increase their effectiveness and ease pressure on their supervisors by assessing where their team is on these dimensions

1. Orientation Stage
   - Members are eager to get started.
   - Members have positive expectations.
   - Energy is spent on attacking the problem in a positive manner.
   - Members look for ways to improve their skills.

2. Dissatisfaction Stage
   - Members may become frustrated.
   - Problems presented to the team may not be easily solved.
   - Members may become angry towards the goals and tasks of the team and toward other team members.
   - Sometimes team members feel incompetent.
   - Energy is focused on redefining members' tasks in a more achievable manner.

3. Resolution Stage
   - Frustration dissipates somewhat.
   - Expectations and reality become more closely meshed.
   - Team member skills are increased.
   - Personal satisfaction is increased.
   - Self-esteem is heightened.

4. Production Stage
   - Members once again become eager to be a part of the team effort.
   - Leadership becomes shared.
   - Members feel greater autonomy.
   - A sense of mutual interdependence with other team members develops.

5. Termination Stage
   - Members feel sad because of ending team relationships.
   - Members often feel a strong sense of accomplishment.

FIGURE 3.4. Developmental stages of an intervention assistance team. From Stokes (1982, p. 12). Copyright 1982 by The Council for Exceptional Children. Reprinted by permission.

and then working with their team to improve to the level of the performing stage. This may mean including a regular examination of team functioning in the team's meeting agenda, setting aside a separate block of time to examine team dynamics via group discussion, role playing, problem-solving sessions, and so on.

Factors in Team Effectiveness

Sundstrom et al. (1990) emphasized other key factors in team effectiveness. These include the *organizational context* and *team boundaries*.

The Organizational Context

The organizational context comprises the "culture" of the organization, the design of the task, the clarity of the team's mission, team autonomy, performance feedback to the team, rewards, training, and physical environment.

According to Sundstrom, a *culture* (a complex set of attitudes) that favors innovation tends to foster team effectiveness. We know that schools tend not to foster innovation but prefer regularity (Sarason, 1982). Consultants need to encourage their supervisors to work for innovative approaches through school channels, so that teams can be encouraged to function better and be freer to consult. Innovative ideas have to address the various needs of supervisors if they are to have a chance even to get off the ground.

Another key factor in team effectiveness is *task design*. Task design takes into account how independently each team member can work or, conversely, how *inter*dependent each member is. On some special services teams, each member (psychologist, social worker, learning consultant) has defined tasks but cannot decide without the full team whether a student should be determined eligible for special education services. Ysseldyke (1984) stressed how psychologists (though this could be applied to any consultant) are often looked to for the final answers on a team decision. The psychologist may enjoy the reinforcement of having people turn to him or her for guidance, but should be aware that this can be a trap. For a team to be truly effective, each member must share equally in the decision making. It may be possible for special services personnel to consult without the help of their team, but the coordination of the various experts can make consultation more effective.

Mission clarity involves having a clearly defined purpose for the team, for example, completing 50 reevaluations a year. Such clarity is not easy to achieve when consultation is the goal, but it can often be defined in such specific ways as reducing dropouts or discipline referrels by a certain percentage. Consultants could look at the numbers of staff served and/or the percentage of staff consulted with (Zins, 1992). Clarity also refers to the time and pace at which something has to be done. Working with the supervisor to define mission clarity can make the team's job easier, can more clearly specify the consultation focus, and can help the supervisor evaluate the consultant's efforts. A good general reference on consultation effectiveness is Gresham and Noell (1992).

Another key factor in team effectiveness is *autonomy*. The degree of autonomy a team has is determined by the role assigned to the leader, if there is a leader. Our child study teams once had leaders, but because of union contract issues, the teams currently operate leaderless and report monthly to the child study team supervisor. Even if a formal leader is not appointed, most teams have individuals who tend to take the lead and set the tone for the group. A team leader can play a role ranging from manager to facilitator and spokesperson to director. Sundstrom et al. (1990) report that self-management can be fostered if leaders act as "unleaders" (Manz & Sims, cited in Sundstrom et al., 1990), that is, if they refuse to be directive and encourage the rest of the team to be involved in sharing leadership. Self-management does not automatically guarantee increased opportunities for consultation, but by implication, it should open up opportunities for such role expansion if teams are so inclined.

Timely *feedback* and *rewards* (including team celebrations) can improve team performance. Look at the rewards the team receives or gives itself. Are they sufficient? Tucker (1981) claimed that school psychologists are often *punished* for finding alternatives to giving students special education services, and rewarded only for determining that students do have special education needs. Therefore, work with the supervisor is critical to reframing the reward system so that consultation becomes recognized.

Training is also important for team functioning, for example in the ways that the team relates to each other, and how they handle various team tasks. Sundstrom et al. (1990) state that little is known about what makes team training programs good, but they recommend teaching a kind of "unleadership" (p. 124) (citing Manz & Sims, 1987). "Unleadership" requires the leader to be able to encourage leadership in all group members. Such training is often absent in the top-down bureaucracies of large school systems.

Finally, Sundstrom et al. (1990) list *physical environment* as a factor that can encourage or inhibit team communication and cohesion. Is the team housed together, and is the seating such that communication is easy? Does the team have a place to meet for conferencing? Teams also need physical barriers if they are to do solitary activities such as write reports or do personal planning. Our special services team is in a large room with the members in close proximity to each other, so communication is easy. However, the room is quite open to students and teachers. This has the advantage of accessibility, but the location makes it hard to do work that requires privacy. However, accessibility is a key factor in fostering consultation with school staff, so that working with the supervisor to promote such accessibility may be a worthwhile goal. Some of our teams are not housed at all in schools, and this lack of accessibility does inhibit consultation.

There is also the human factor of inertia, which might make it easier for a consultant to do write-ups at a comfortable desk at the central administration building far from the school instead of pushing him/herself to drive to the school and do consulting outreach to school staff. Examine physical surroundings and see whether they can be modified to be more accessible for consulting. If they are not easily modifiable, the team may have to locate itself at specified times where members are more accessible to school staff (e.g., faculty lounges).

The above issues affect how well a team performs. They need to be considered by teams and supervisors when consulting tasks are planned. Sundstrom's group notes that effective team members often develop overlapping roles even if they have a clear team mission. They also are often characterized by decentralized communication and "unleadership" (flexible, rotating leadership), which appears to work better with "teams faced with unpredictable inputs or uncertain outcomes" (Sundstrom et al., 1990, p. 123). The implications for working with supervisors are to help them become aware of such research so as to help with team development, and to use this information to see what can be done to change team roles, clarify the team's mission, and so on.

Team Boundaries

Boundaries specify how integrated the team is into its surroundings and how differentiated (specialized) it is. Supervisors may unwittingly inhibit consultation effectiveness by not looking more closely at team boundaries. In our school system, teams that were too differentiated were seen as outsiders by the teaching staff, who felt they had little in common with the team members. One result of this perception was that the teachers' union (to which the special services teams belonged) was unresponsive to the teams' needs. This problem was solved using two different strategies. First, the teams attempted to break down boundaries by encouraging more special services team participation in union meetings and functions. Second, uniting the teams (increasing differentiation from the other departments) to create a massed vote for an opposing union during an election also got the attention of the existing union. Although the incumbent union won the election, union members began to recognize the special services teams as a power with which to be reckoned. While this example does not have direct implications for supervisors, it illustrates the image problem special services teams may have. Supervisors need to be made continually aware of how team boundaries get in the way of staff acceptance and effective consultation.

The Problem of Categorizing Special Services Teams

Sundstrom et al., after describing what makes for an effective team, then describe the four types of teams they have observed, according to such criteria as the following: how differentiated each team is (i.e., unique academic qualifications or training); whether they work on long or short chronological cycles; whether they require brief, high-level performance or longer-term repeated, continuous tasks; and whether they have a high or low level of integration (i.e., tend to work with others or by themselves).

The team types are the following:

1. *Advice/involvement* (advisory committees, boards, quality control circles)
2. *Production/service* (assembly crews, data processing groups, flight attendant crews, maintenance crews)
3. *Project development* (research and planning teams)
4. *Action/negotiation* (sports teams, entertainment groups, surgery teams, cockpit groups)

Sundstrom's review demonstrates vividly a problem special teams face, because the typical special services team does not fit his taxonomy. Rather, the special services teams I have observed tend to have characteristics in common with all four categories of teams that Sundstrom and Altman (1989) list.

Special services teams often have the high differentiation (specialists who are experts) characteristic of groups 3 and 4. These teams also range in function from a low integration level characteristic of groups 1 and 3 (much work by themselves) to the high integration of groups 2 and 4 (great deal of contact and involvement with clients). Special services personnel work at a low integration level when they are writing reports, and at high integration functions when coordinating with others over meeting special education evaluation deadlines, synchronizing work with teachers when they are consulting with them, or arranging a counseling schedule so that students are not taken out of the same class period every day.

Special services teams have work cycles that can be brief or long, as occurs in group 1. This occurs when members serve on school committees if they want to have an impact at consultation Level III or IV, or when their own consultation functions, like that of my team, are experimental. Yet, much of special services team work is also repeated or continuous, a characteristic of group 2. This includes regular cycles of reevaluating students or holding reviews of IEPs. On the other hand, another work cycle variation involves brief performance events under new conditions requiring immediate creativity and innovation. Group 4, which includes surgical and athletic teams, which have to respond to unpredictable events quickly, illustrates this cycle. However, the crisis intervention often demanded of special services teams with hostile or suicidal students certainly requires this same kind of improvisation.

In view of this broad range of special services team functions, Sundstrom's research, which relates boundaries or types of supervision to effective output in each of the four types of teams he discusses, may be difficult to apply to special services teams. We can, however, see how varied and challenging the task of special services teams is, and we can draw the following conclusions: It is clear that special services teams need to be accessible yet have time and the physical environment (space) to do solitary writing and planning work. They need boundaries to practice their specialties and assert their importance, yet those boundaries should be permeable enough to relate to other staff as insiders, not outsiders. They need a clear task design, balancing their independent work with the cooperative demands of a team. Teams require a clear mission or goal, and they must function with a reasonable degree of autonomy if creativity in meeting school problems and challenges is to be cultivated. Teams should receive appropriate feedback and rewards. Special services teams need to make decisions as to how integrated with the school they will be, and what the ideal work cycles will be.

These are all issues for teams to work out with each other and to negotiate with their supervisors. Also, teams can examine how effectively they work and relate to each other using some of the ideas of Reddin (cited in Sergiovanni & Starratt, 1988; see Chapter 4). By focusing on some of the issues cited above, consultants will have a clearer idea of how best to organize their team for effective functioning. This will, in turn, make the consultant's relationship with his/her supervisor much more productive.

Implementing Teaming to Help the Supervisor

One way to learn any concept is to practice it. Why not consider doing inservice programs for other teams in the area of team functioning?

Such programs could include lectures on the basic team functioning issues spelled out in the work of Tuckman (1965), Stokes (1982), Maher and Bennett (1984), Hamway and Elias (1988), and Sundstrom et al. (1990). Lectures could be followed by small group discussions analyzing each team according to which categories of Sundstrom and Altman (1989) best fit it and deciding to which stage of team development it has progressed. Although it is difficult to categorize an entire special services team using just one of Sundstrom's criteria, the attempt to do so should be illuminating. (For instance, you may decide your team is most like the production/service team because of the bulk of team time spent on reevaluating special education students.) Sharing of each groups' conclusions could then take place, providing emotional support from the other groups' experiences. Groups could then set goals for next steps (clarify mission, increase integration, reduce boundaries, etc.). Goals could include adding functions of the other Sundstrom group types. For example, a group more typical of the production/service group might decide to emulate group 4, the action/negotiation team, and help the school with suicide or violence prevention and intervention efforts. They would then have to increase their level of integration and change their work cycle to be more responsive to crises. Brainstorming sessions could be conducted in subsequent small group meetings.

Such efforts will help the supervisor and will also prepare teams to be more effective as consultants. Sundstrom noted the effects of training and consultation in helping teams to function better but said that little evidence exists about the proper design of such programs. Kuehnel and Kuehnel (cited in Alpert & Meyers, 1983) listed 13 areas in which consultants should be trained, but they did not specify whether these should be used for training *teams*. West and Cannon (1988) at the University of Texas–Austin recommended training for consultants in such skills as interpersonal communication, empathic potential, ability to tolerate differences of opinion, being calm in crises, having a positive self-concept, doing collaborative problem solving, and being able to evaluate effectiveness of consultation. They too did not specify these areas for effective *team* functioning, but consultants might try to translate these individual skills into teamwork applications. These applications could range from trying to build team members' self-concepts to evaluating the effectiveness of team efforts at consulting or other functions.

Hamway and Elias (1988, citing Stokes, 1982) provide a checklist of team skills required to do consultation (Figure 3.3). I suggest that consultants evaluate their skills as team members on this list, and prepare to fill any gaps they find. Such a list can provide a basis for discussion on the team's meeting agenda. Why not talk in team meetings about such issues as instructional strategies, sequences of academic content areas, or how to develop collaborative consultation skills? Every team should meet regularly and have on its agenda a discussion item dealing with team relationships and skills. Consultants should know the areas in which their team needs further development. Certainly, improving team functioning is a worthwhile goal in itself. Work with the supervisor to develop good training programs to enhance team effectiveness.

This chapter concerned meeting the needs of the supervisor. We have looked at team members' reactions to supervisors, and how such reactions color the supervisor–supervisee relationship. The motives and needs, worries, and pressures of supervisors have been explored as they apply to special services fields and how these motives affect consultants' ability to function freely to do consultation. Methods of helping the supervisor succeed while meeting such needs were discussed. Finally, team self-diagnosis and functioning were connected to the team–supervisor relationship. Helping teams become more effective is an important way to make the job of the supervisor easier and thereby to remove another possible block to consultation entry.

4

The Teachers

Sanction from the supervisor and the principal is a necessary but not sufficient condition for the success of consultation. Once the consultant has achieved sanction to consult, he or she is likely to find that the most frequent consultee is the teacher (Meyers's Levels II and III) (Parsons & Meyers, 1984; Meyers et al., 1979). Consultation with teachers is crucial because, when effective, it leads to more holistic consultation resulting in schoolwide programming, Meyers's Level IV.

In this chapter I present my thoughts and experiences regarding elements of the school's culture and climate that affect consultation entry with teachers, the various teacher groups that need to be involved if entry is to be achieved, and how to attend to teachers' needs and pressures. I argue for creating a performance investment for teachers so they will feel an ownership of the procedures used by the special services team. This ownership makes teachers perform not just routinely, but because they feel invested in what they are doing at the levels of Maslow's needs for esteem and self-actualization. I explore the special services team's role in smoothing teacher relationships with administrators and look at Meyers's levels of consultation as they relate to the task of easing the burdens teachers face.

THE SCHOOL CULTURE

The eager consultant, anxious to implement the project, may at times resemble the bull in the china shop. Like the bull, the consultant may move ahead without noticing the surroundings—especially the school culture—confident in his/her professional knowledge and anxious to teach teachers how to teach more effectively. Of course, most teachers already know how to teach, and even if they are in need of help because they are burned out or working in a district that has many problems, their talents are still there, though perhaps buried in discouragement. The effective consultant approaches the teacher with a great deal of respect, regardless of any perceived lacks of deficits in the teacher's functioning. However, individual respect is not sufficient for effective consultation entry. The consultant must also be aware that each teacher, besides being a member of a profession with its own norms, roles, language, and body of knowledge, is a member of an *organizational* culture (Caplan, 1970).

Therefore, the special services staff person who wants to consult must become aware of the behaviors that characterize the teaching profession in the particular culture. The organizational culture refers to the culture of the specific school and district, which has its own characteristics, some similar and some rather different from those of the teaching profession. The teaching profession also has similarities to and differences from the consultant's own profession, even if the consultant formerly was a teacher. (I have already discussed the problems a principal has when promoted from the position of teacher.)

If the consultant is from the outside, perhaps from a university or a mental health center, the organizational norms of the school may be drastically different from the consultant's regular work setting. (For example, research is valued little in the public schools, in contrast to its almost sacred value in the university setting.) The consultant must be prepared to become a part of the school culture (Sarason, 1982), though Newman (1967) cautioned that the role of guest might be more appropriate for the consultant. Newman and Sarason were outside consultants. My guess is that Sarason, whose work is more recent, found a more flexible role for the consultant than might have existed 15 years earlier. My own preference is to start in the school as a guest and later become part of what I hope is an expanded culture, more open to change.

All schools have a culture, a set of norms and behaviors, expectations, and values, which provides teachers, and others, with a sense of stability and belonging. Not knowing these values can be as disastrous as, for instance, back slapping and insisting on shaking hands with Asian business people. Cultural norms can include appropriate body language, personal space, or level of formality (Caplan, 1970). For example, the custom in our schools is to address everyone by Ms., Mr., and Dr., rather than by first names. Male teachers usually wear a shirt and tie, all our assemblies begin with the Pledge of Allegiance and the National Anthem, and nobody risks taking time up by asking questions if a faculty meeting runs late.

Cultural Regularities

Sarason (1982) called the most important of these norms "regularities," which must be documented and thoroughly understood by the consultant in order for entry to occur and consultation to be successful. As noted in earlier chapters, a regularity might be a state program for determining reading level with a standardized test, a classroom where the norm is for students to listen and not ask questions, or a 3-day-a-week physical education program. The outcome of each custom is not always what was originally intended when the program or schedule was planned. The consultant needs to look at any discrepancies between these regularities and their intended outcomes and recognize that in most school cultures there is no procedure built in to evaluate such discrepancies. For example, do 4 years of 5-days-a-week high school English really accomplish the district's goal of improving student communication skills? Cultures tend to ignore the many alternatives that exist for school regularities, yet if changes are to occur in the culture, the existing regularities may have to be changed to produce new outcomes. Sarason asserts that most attempts to make changes in schools ignore these regularities and, as such, are doomed to failure. The consultant, therefore, must identify the school regularities if the school culture is to be understood and changed. The consultant has the challenge of becoming a catalyst to create new cultures open to change (Adams & Spencer, 1986).

The school culture is bigger than any individual. Creative teachers may find themselves caught in a school culture that fosters rigidity and conformity. Rigidity, for example, might cause teachers to resist sharing classroom management problems with principals or colleagues. An overly conforming culture might discourage teachers from teaching more than one subject (e.g., a math teacher teaching history of math or a science teacher teaching science fiction and relating it to the development of scientific concepts). Many school cultures deter teachers from going beyond their "specialty," and dissuade them from doing things outside the classroom as well, such as relating to parents, community, and other sources of help for children. Such cultures tend to discourage creativity and the change that often results from it. Flexible teachers and consultants who want to look objectively at the value of certain school regularities in such a setting will often find themselves frustrated by powerful resistance from staff. On the other hand, a more liberal culture, oriented to parent and student input into the curriculum, that focuses on teaching values and problem solving as opposed to basic academic skills, may resist the objective measurement and recording necessary for effective consultation (Gagne, 1977; Kratochwill & Van Someren, 1985).

School culture can dictate that special services teams serve only as testers or as removers of troublesome students from the classroom (i.e., a culture of individual diagnosis) (Newman, 1967). A regularity for counselors may be that they counsel disruptive students but do not consult with teachers or principals, because their "place" is not in the classroom except to do group guidance (another regularity).

Professional Preciousness

Cultural values in a school may reinforce "professional preciousness" (Sarason et al., 1966), that is, a belief that one's own professional skills are unique. Such values exaggerate the differences between the professions. Caplan (cited by Erchul, 1991) urged that consultants respect the autonomy and competence of consultees of other professions. Johnson et al. (1988), however, noted instead that regular education teachers view themselves as inferior in knowledge to special education teachers and therefore view them (in the consulting role) as superior. Gallesich (1973) identified this as a trap for consultants, whom the culture may perceive as miracle workers and therefore scapegoats for school disasters or excuses to sanction the firing of a teacher. Sometimes special education departments view counselors as unknowledgeable about the particular problems a special education child has, whereas the counseling department may have the preconception that special education lacks the ability to plan vocationally for its students. Sarason et al. (1966) give the example of how each department becomes its own enclave, where communication is better within the department than across departmental lines. Such departments only see the "piece" of the child that is their responsibility and cannot look objectively at the needs of the whole child. Such views limit the growth of knowledge within these departments and stimulate competition between them.

Sarason (1982) suggests a solution whereby various professionals, across departments, take responsibility for managing a case (with, of course, the freedom to call in a specialist if they need that help) in order to give each the big picture. In our high school, we decided that a counselor, coach, and school psychologist would jointly manage the case of an athletically talented graduating special education student who had a severe learning disability. He wanted to go to college to play basketball and had been offered a number of scholarships. Unfortunately, the colleges that wanted him did not have learning disabilities support systems. The coach was unaware of the extent of the student's academic deficit until he was filled in by the school psychologist. The school psychologist, who was the student's case manager, was unaware of the coach's college plans. The school psychologist researched colleges that did offer adequate supports, the coach determined whether those schools offered the appropriate athletic opportunities, and he and the counselor worked to expedite the applications. All three professionals helped the student with various aspects of the college application. None of the individual professionals had the big picture until they conferred together, dropping the customary boundaries.

Culture and Teacher Isolation

One common aspect of school culture is the expectation that teachers should be able to handle their problems themselves, without consultation or a team or case study approach (Sarason et al., 1966; Rosenfield, 1987). In one study of self-contained classrooms, few teachers of behaviorally disordered children sought help from regular education teachers (their own colleagues), although they were willing to seek out the school psychologist (McManus & Kauffman, 1991). Rosenfield notes that teachers who ask for help fear that the helper perceives them as incompetant (and some helpers also share this view). There is a fine line between encouraging teachers to ask for help and Shore and Vieland's (1989) recommendation to support teachers' roles as "executives" in their classroom. Rosenfield (1987) also encourages teachers to solve problems within the classroom context and tries to increase their control. Sarason (1988) said that consultants should work toward encouraging more teacher teamwork and collaboration to reduce their isolation so that participatory problem solving can take place (see also Ponti et al., 1988; Hyman & Dougherty, 1988). One of the keys to penetrating the school culture is to work with *groups* of teachers (Sergiovanni & Starratt, 1988) because that is where the dimensions of culture are shaped. Here the complex coalitions and sources of power that make organizations harder to enter become more accessible.

Some school cultures are based on a "production ethic" (Sarason, 1982) in which academic achievement is valued over skills of living and surviving in a diverse community. Rosenfield (1987) states that the teacher's need to get through the curriculum (rather than having students master the material) is a strong cultural value that poses an obstacle to the consultant. Sarason (1982) claims that such cultural values often come from the demands of parents and community, as well as from administrators.

The consultant's *own* culture influences how the consultant views the school, and the consultant must be constantly aware of his/her biases about what schools should be. The consultant's ideas of what constitutes individual worth and how that relates to achievement may be very different from those of the teachers or students with whom the consultant is working. If, for example, the consultant greatly values a college education, and the teachers he/she works with have to prepare students for vocational-level or semiskilled jobs, his/her own expectations may interfere with the consultation he/she attempts. Sarason (1982) suggests that a consultant needs to assess his/her own abilities if the consultant wishes to help others improve theirs (see Chapter 3).

Culture and Faculty–Student Communication

Culture also comprises norms for communication between students and faculty (Gallesich, 1973). At one school in our district, which had poor communication between staff and students, certain staff members viewed students as if they were inmates of a prison. There are many such schools (Sergiovanni & Starratt, 1988), often called "custodial schools" (Willower, Eidell, & Hoy, 1967), at which students are rigidly controlled, do not participate in decision making, and are expected to accept decisions without question. They are viewed as irresponsible, undisciplined, and untrustworthy, and punitive methods for control are often the norm. When I proposed to a group of teachers that students be included on a committee to help improve discipline and student behavior, one teacher commented, "You don't ask the prisoners how to run the prison, do you?" While enlightened educators and consultants might be horrified by such an attitude, ignoring it could sabotage any consultation efforts. Instead, a consultant in the meeting used the guerrilla tactic of finding out what this teacher's agenda was, exploring his values, and obtaining suggestions.

The teacher had been at the school many years, had seen many demographic and racial changes, and was having difficulty adapting to the present group of students. He was concerned about the students' lack of discipline and respect for teachers and demanded the old-line respect for elders that one sees little of these days. He could not understand how including such students could be helpful. His opinions were representative of those of many of the staff at that school.

During this meeting, I chose not to argue with this cynical teacher but instead delved for other teachers' views in order to obtain a balance. The discussion ended with at least some of the teachers asserting a more positive view of the same group of students. They expressed their view that student participation *was* important.

Here the culture was one that supported repression and authoritarianism. The first step in opening this culture to change was to provide an opportunity for teachers to speak their minds, so that the cynic would not perceive the entire group as supportive of his views. The consultant was perceived as someone opening up opportunities for dialogue, and hence a step toward entry was achieved. Such a step would be at Level III of Meyers's consultation approach because it began to change a teacher. It also was a beginning at Level IV because it opened a teacher dialogue and suggested the possibility of school programming to further expand that dialogue. Some of these teachers did not believe students could contribute positively to improving the school, especially in areas in which authority had reigned. The consultant's guerrilla tactic was to build more trust between students and teachers, for example, by having students model responsible behavior.

Changing the school culture involves a change in trust level between teachers and students. At this junior high school, the consultant identified the "worst students" in the school by picking out the class section with the most frequent discipline referrals. This classroom, coincidentally, was also the lowest-achieving regular education class in the school. Via a group counseling approach welcomed by the teachers because it took place in the classroom (relieving them of some of the management pressure), students were trained to orient the incoming seventh graders as to how to succeed in junior high. This project was chosen because seventh graders were viewed as the most problematic group in the school. The students in this class first had to verbalize which behaviors would produce school success, which all were able to do despite their own failure records, and then rehearse what to say to the sixth graders, including advice on effective behaviors in adapting to junior high school life.

Next, trips to feeder elementary schools were organized by the consultant, helped by the good relationships previously established with those principals. On the day of the trip, the students were groomed much better than usual, were nicely dressed, and comported themselves quite well when speaking to an auditorium full of sixth graders. The increased status they received back at the junior high school among peers was remarkable. Peers admired their dress and grooming. They expressed envy that our students got to be emissaries to other elementary schools and wanted to know how they could get to do that too. The teachers began to feel more of a sense of trust and respect for these students. Improved entry opportunities were achieved by the consultant because he was perceived as not afraid to work with the most difficult students.

This example illustrates attempts at entry using Meyers's Levels I (group and individual counseling), II and III (work with teacher on group techniques and attitude change), and IV (obtaining sanction from principals to orient incoming seventh graders).

Changing Teacher Expectations

The consultant can enter the culture of a school through teachers' recreational activities. The smart consultant will participate in these activities. At one school, I did not really break through to the staff until I played in a softball game at the school picnic. In enthusiastically fielding a ball, I fell over a teacher while tagging that teacher out. This effort placed me in a role other than professional expert, and though the staff respected me for that expert role, sharing an activity valued by staff, and at a physical level, placed me in a new light. I also brought my daughter to the picnic. Sharing part of my personal life with the teachers also was meaningful. It changed the "distant expert" role into one of family man like the rest of the staff.

Martin (Meyers et al., 1979) noted the referent power that comes from being in an authority role. Here people admire the consultant because of his/her title and their desire to identify with the consultant. Johnson et al. (1988) agreed that the consultant is often seen as superior. This stereotype of miracle worker (Gallesich, 1973) needs to be challenged. Showing a human side is one way to achieve entry into the teachers' culture.

Broadening Teachers' Perspectives

So far, we have discussed cultures that believe in narrow staff roles, cultures in which departments become their own enclaves, those that discourage teachers from seeking help, and cultures that overstress academic achievement and dictate only narrow ways in which staff and students can communicate. A school's culture may reflect other values, such as expecting the same degree of mastery from every student. This cultural norm suggests that it is undemocratic for some students to get more help or attention than others. This makes it hard for the consultant to individualize an academic or behavior management program for a student. The culture often pressures teachers to raise academic levels rather than help students with what they *need* to learn (Rosenfield, 1987; Sarason, 1982).

Sarason (1982) urged consultants to support teachers who are willing to relate to students outside the limited sphere of the classroom. A teacher needs to become a real mentor to do this. This means that teachers, whether of math, art, or science, are willing to work on anything a student needs, from study skills, problem solving, or reading skills to developing a real relationship with the student or his/her parents. Yet the culture of schools often says otherwise, by delimiting the functions of a teacher. Finding ways to relate the consultation to these cultural values is critical.

Holistic consultation requires that the special services team or outside consultant consider means of individualizing programs to better serve the needs of students. The consultant needs to help staff realize that individual change and confidence building with students will, in the long run, further the school's goals of meeting curriculum requirements. The holistic approach posits the necessity of working not only with teachers to accomplish this, but also with principals and administrators so that support from above can facilitate the teachers' efforts. This may require the consultant to find research data to show how an individualized approach can facilitate the achievement of academic goals. Success at promoting individualization can change the culture because it shows how valuing the individual helps student morale, increases teacher success, and also makes for climate changes at the school.

Sarason (1982) also recognized that every teacher cannot like every student. Teachers should not feel guilty if they cannot relate well to all students assigned to them. Our team often recommended class reassignment because of personality clashes between students and teachers. However, we often ran into cultural values opposed to this. We were accused of not training students for the realities of life—of learning to get along with a great variety of people.

Many school cultures emphasize educating people for society's purposes, and as such they are group oriented. This view is in opposition to psychology's need to look at the individual. If the consultant is a psychologist or counselor, his/her graduate school training is likely to have been individual focused. Hence, in many school settings the consultant needs to make the adjustment to a culture that does not value the individual nearly as much as the group.

Consultation with such a group-oriented culture must encourage greater individualization. This may involve encouraging teachers to bring out more from each student, increasing creativity and critical thinking, increasing student reliability or responsibility (societal values that schools are "supposed to" teach, and therefore this may be supported by the culture), or developing peer support groups in the classroom for increased production.

In peer support groups, stronger students are rewarded for work with weaker students. Much work is currently being done on student-oriented work responsibility where those in the classroom become responsible for their learning and that of their peers. Slavin's (1990) work (cited in Moses, 1991a) with "detracking" schools is an attempt to provide greater individualization while mixing bright, average, and below-average students and having them engage in cooperative learning. They work together in small groups and are responsible for making sure that everyone in the group learns the material. The brighter students find that their understanding of the material is reinforced when they help slower students. Although each student is tested individually for his/her knowledge, the group is rewarded for the performance of the slower individuals. Such programs are good for breaking into a culture that is group oriented, as they make clear that the whole group benefits when needy students receive the help they require.

Brown, Campione, and Palincsar's work with reciprocal teaching (cited in Moses, 1991b) also encourages individual skill building through a method that minimizes disruption of (the culture of) normal classroom functioning. Here, students in a reading group take turns as discussion leader to go over material in the book being read. They must practice four strategies: questioning, clarifying text, summarizing, and predicting upcoming events. These strategies are typically not used by students with learning problems yet are often a normal part of a successful student's repertoire. The teacher guides discussion, but does not lead it, and supports the students who are leading at the moment. The disruption is minimal because the essential structure of the reading group task stays the same. It is still the same reading group, and the class schedule does not have to change.

In another study by Brown in 1988 (cited in Moses, 1991b), fifth and sixth graders researched a topic, wrote about it, and illustrated it using a computer, and each student became the expert on one section of the material. These "experts" had to teach the material and prepare test questions on it. Here, the classroom teacher must give up some authority, thereby disrupting the classroom culture more than did the previous approach. This might be a difficult task (Sarason, 1982) in school cultures where student input is not valued, but if the consultant shares data showing that students who teach others also improve their own achievement, this cultural barrier might be lowered.

Other schemas could include encouraging parental support for teacher goals or sharing clinical diagnostic data about a student and encouraging the teacher to develop means of tackling the academic deficits. Essentially, in this approach, the consultant intervenes to change the culture to focus more on the individual by demonstrating that the culture's larger goals of group advancement can be met via attention to individual needs.

At one of our inner-city elementary schools with a primarily minority population, the culture was oriented rigidly toward increasing standardized achievement test scores (often leaving far behind many of the academically deficient students whom consultants are called in to help). The consultant, who personally disliked such use of achievement tests, agreed to help the school raise test scores, thereby joining with the cultural values of the school. He worked with the special services team and teachers (see similar work by Knight et al., 1981) to increase language stimulation in the classroom and at home (based on a review of past data showing that language and vocabulary were among the lowest of the achievement test scores). The issue here is that the consultant took the *culture* into account in deciding where to intervene yet used established approaches to help students develop skills, such as working with teachers to increase student verbalization by asking questions and creating discussion opportunities (Liddle, cited in Magary, 1967; Sarason, 1982), involving parents in a program of increasing language stimulation at home, and so on. The culture, because it valued test results, was open to an intervention that might have a positive effect on those results. Hence, the consultant must design interventions around the cultural needs, keeping in mind that if there is success, the culture may be more open to change. Here the change might be classroom emphasis on language, moving away from rote preparation to pass a standardized test.

THE SCHOOL CLIMATE

Climate is different from culture in that it describes an *atmosphere* at a particular school. Regularities (part of school culture, not climate) tend to be more stable *across many* schools. Climate is an enduring characteristic of a *particular* school created by the *leadership,* usually the principal. It includes atmosphere, working conditions, job demands, and so forth. In contrast, culture is more a function of the staff, although it can also reflect collective administrative values and norms. A climate can be open or closed (Sergiovanni & Starratt, 1988) in terms of its receptivity to ideas, respect for individual needs, staff spirit, and the general degree of rigidity of practice.

Climate as a Function of Management Style

Climate can be likened to a management system (Likert, 1967), of which Likert identified four types:

1. Exploitative–authoritarian
2. Benevolent–authoritarian
3. Consultative
4. Participative

System 1 leadership (exploitative–authoritarian) has no confidence in subordinates, motivating them through the use of physical security, economic needs, and status. This leadership has no understanding of the problems of its subordinates and the infrequent interaction it has with subordinates in characterized by fear and distrust. Subordinates have no input into decision making, and the goals set by the administration are usually resisted by the subordinates. Control exists only at the top.

System 2 (benevolent–authoritarian) principals show a condescending confidence in their staff and do show more concern for status, affiliation, and achievement needs. They have some awareness of the problems of subordinates but still little interaction with them. As in System 1, they never involve staff in decisions, although they sometimes consult them. Control and goals still come mainly from the top. Systems 1 and 2 most closely fit Sergiovanni and Starratt's (1988) description of a closed climate.

System 3 leadership (consultative) still controls decisions but has much more confidence and trust in staff and is willing to offer them new experiences in addition to satisfying basic economic and ego needs. System 3 leaders have a good understanding of the problems of staff and moderate levels of interaction with them, often with a fair amount of confidence and trust. Staff are often consulted about decisions but are still rarely involved in decision making. Control, while still at the top, is shared with middle levels of management and to some degree at lower levels.

The participative system, 4, comes closest to Sergiovanni and Starratt's (1988) open climate. Here leadership has complete trust in subordinates and seeks to motivate them by trying to meet the entire range of human needs. They understand the problems of staff, have extensive interaction with them on a friendly basis, and make sure that staff are fully involved in decision making. High organizational goals are sought by all levels of the school hierarchy. Often the lower levels of a participative climate press for even higher goals and organizational controls than do the upper levels.

Measuring Climate

Climate can be measured by various techniques, for example, the Organizational Climate Description Questionnaire developed by Halpin and Croft (Halpin, 1967), and its revision (Hoy & Clover, 1986) from Rutgers University. The latter describes the school climate in terms of three dimensions of principal behavior (supportive, directive, and restrictive) and three dimensions of teacher behavior that is reactive to the principal (collegial, intimate, and disengaged). The supportive principal has sincere concern for teachers. The directive principal's supervisory style is rigid and close, while the restrictive principal hinders teacher's work through paper work, committee requirements, and other duties that interfere with teaching responsibilities. Collegial teacher behavior shows pride in one's professionality, enthusiasm, and respect for colleagues. Intimate teacher behavior reflects strong social networks, with many teachers as close personal friends who support each other. The disengaged teacher feels a lack of meaning and is just putting in time, demonstrating nonproductive behavior that is often negative and critical.

Gottfredson and Hollifield (1988) discuss how to measure school climate, including the use of the Effective School Battery (Gottfredson, n.d.) which describes students' and teachers' perceptions about school climate, measuring 34 indicators of effective school performance.

The Work Environment Scale (Insel & Moos, 1974) is a 90-item questionnaire given to teachers and administrators. It measures physical and psychological conditions at a work setting and is a good measure of teacher satisfaction or dissatisfaction. Items reflect how supervisors treat employees, how free the work atmosphere is, and how open people can be.

The Pennsylvania Department of Education (n.d.) developed a School Climate Survey (Appendix B) which can be given to students, teachers, parents, and administrators. It measures General Climate Factors (respect), Program Determinants (individualization, program flexibility), Process Determinants (examining alternatives, resolving conflicts), and Material Determinants (staffing, salaries, physical plant). The subject rates how the current situation is and also what it should be.

I believe consultants who use such measures to assess the climate of the school will be much more effective in achieving entry, although Hyman and Dougherty (1988) doubted the utility of such instruments, favoring a closer look at the *process* of measuring climate instead.

School principals may be open to measuring climate if they are having problems with student or teacher morale. They may be interested in research that shows that a more open climate makes for higher test achievement and better student behavior and attendance (e.g., Rutter, Maughan, Mortimer, & Ouston, 1979). In such a climate, teachers have better attitudes toward learning, praise students more, and involve students as active learners.

Climate Descriptors and the Consultant

The results of a climate survey should highlight for consultants and special services personnel points of entry and areas in which to exercise caution. For example, entering a school in which the teacher behavior is characterized as intimate (Hoy & Clover, 1986) suggests that it may be difficult to break into the tight teacher social networks because the teachers see the consultant as an intruder. Working with teachers who are disengaged means dealing with burnout and setting realistic goals. The consultant attempting entry with teachers in a climate in which, for example, hindrance factors loom large (e.g., excessive paper work), will need to employ consultation methods that take little of a teacher's time or use a more holistic approach (Meyers's Level IV) to change administrative policies in order to diminish hindrance factors. Climate measures may open the eyes of principals who were not aware of how they were restricting staff functioning, or how they could tune in better to the needs of a disengaged staff. The more rigid principal will resist such measures, and the consultant may have to attempt entry around that principal's priorities first (Chapter 2).

If the staff is disengaged, they may be as much at fault as the principal for not being involved in the planning. The consultant needs to help staff be more assertive when dealing with principals, so that they ask clearly for what they want. This may mean enlisting the aid of the more influential teachers (Roth, 1980), helping teachers to increase their sense of mastery (Caplan, 1970), and improving their skills in dealing with organizations (Schmuck, cited in Alpert & Meyers, 1983; Schmuck, 1990).

Closed climates can have a palpable denseness to them—a lack of breathing room and a sense of pressure on people. I have walked through school corridors where that closed atmosphere feels like a vise: Where principals, in a futile attempt to encourage high staff achievement and organization, have closed off even the normal greeting of people in the hallway, and teachers have the feeling that they are always being watched. Imagine how it feels to be a teacher in such a setting— what a challenge to the consultant who wants to open up such a climate. As noted in Chapter 2, the consultant must behave as a guest in this setting, follow the rules, and find out the principal's priorities. Consultation may then start to open up along the lines of such priorities as improving the organization of instruction. The consultant's ability to provide support for the teachers who are isolated in such a setting (without being trapped into stimulating a staff rebellion) (Caplan, 1970; Sarason, 1982) is a key to entry. The consultant must maintain a careful balance between the needs of the principal and those of the teacher, but the consultant can influence the climate.

Hoy and Miskel (1987) indicated, for example, that the open climate is characterized by *supportive leadership* and a high degree of *collegial* and *intimate* teacher behavior. Open climates are low in directiveness and restrictiveness from principals and are not characterized by teacher disengagement. The consultant, then, can support an open climate by working to increase collegial and intimate behavior on the part of teachers in part by becoming a model for collegiality and intimacy. To do so, the consultant must build self-esteem in the staff (first finding it in him/herself). This modeling must also produce results for whoever created the closed climate or it may fail to engage the principal in fostering a more open climate.

The consultant can open up such a climate by obtaining sanction from a principal to work with teacher groups to accomplish the principal's goals. Such groups could work on increasing staff achievement or organization, writing staff procedure manuals, or other such activities that seem on the surface to increase the principal's control. However, the *process* involved in such meetings can also stimulate teachers' self-esteem and ownership of school procedures and improve communication among teachers and with the principal. Such a process can achieve at least the collegial aspect of the open climate. The supportive leadership required for an open climate, it is hoped, will come from the consultant's work with the principal (Chapter 2).

THE FOCUS OF INTERVENTION

The successful consultant will step back and look at how staff alliances are formed. For example, teachers can be categorized by their grade-level assignment, age and experience, special interests (union, student group leadership, etc.), or specialty. Each of these gives the teacher something in common with his/her peers and can be utilized by the consultant to tap into the teacher's motives.

Grade-Level Focus

The consultant or special services team member must be aware of the special needs of teachers based on the grade they teach. Kindergarten teachers have priorities very different from those of the third-grade, seventh-grade, or twelfth-grade teacher. Third-grade teachers are concerned with the increased complexity of language skills and vocabulary building, as the difficulty of the material becomes more apparent at that level. Many seventh graders have trouble with the transition from small elementary schools (where essentially they had one teacher most of the day) to a large junior high school with departmentalized programs and many teachers to adjust to. These teachers often become more concerned with behavior issues than do those who teach third grade.

The guerrilla tactic needed here is to mobilize teachers on grade levels by dealing with *their* agendas, Levels III and IV interventions. While typical special services personnel might be concerned with identifying seventh-grade students with learning or behavior problems, the seventh-grade culture and climate themselves may be conducive to problems, and therefore the consultant must tune in to the teachers and deal with that. Again, we need to look at the school via Meyers's Level IV.

At one of my schools, seventh-grade teachers had few chances to meet together except at lunch, where they would either discuss social topics or complain about students or work loads. I made it a point to eat my lunch with these teachers. Their frustration at a departmental system that provided little opportunity to discuss individual students or develop teaching skills prompted me to arrange meetings of all the seventh-grade teachers. The principal, concerned with the high frequency of discipline and special education referrals from grade 7, was glad to have me convene such a meeting. There the teachers could vent their frustration and then get on to the task of improving the educational program.

Our special services team, which serviced three elementary schools, learned that their third-grade teachers had many problems in common. The team prevailed on the principals of these schools to permit interschool meetings of those teachers to discuss and share their problems (see also Wallin & Ferguson, cited in Magary, 1967). The teachers welcomed the meetings, reiterated that they needed the support of their third-grade teacher colleagues (see Ponti et al., 1988), and said that they felt less isolated after attending these meetings.

Enrichment Teachers

Many efforts at school improvement focus on the teachers of the core subjects: English, mathematics, history, and science. Enrichment teachers (health, art, music, physical education, shop, etc.) are seen as ancillary staff, not involved in the "meat and potatoes" of education. The consultant needs to take another look at these teachers, for they can be key allies and often may be enablers or power brokers in the school. More important, they have knowledge and skills that can help regular teachers and they often see students in a different light. For example, art and gym teachers see the hands-on and kinesthetic skills of the students. They see them in larger group settings and in competition using physical and creative, as opposed to academic, skills. One vocational–technical teacher of graphic arts (printing) took special education students with poor math skills and taught them to center material on a page using a grid instead of complex calculations. Many special education students are more visual, preferring this modality to verbal or sequential thinking, so this method was quite suitable for them. Their math teacher might have been surprised at how adept they became at this task.

A special education senior was having trouble completing his work so that he could graduate. His gym teacher, to whom he was close, was instrumental in bringing parents and special services personnel together to resolve the difficulty he was facing. One of the parents was in denial, refusing to recognize that her child was neglecting his work. The gym teacher's influence was sufficient to bring about parental cooperation. A study schedule was developed with specific objectives (Levels I and II). Meyers's Level III also was involved here because the gym teacher needed guidance in clarifying her expectations so the student could know exactly what he had to do to pass. The student was graduated following intensive counseling by the school psychologist and gym teacher (Levels I and II) and counseling parents to provide structure (Level II).

Librarians

Librarians are another kind of specialist with specific skills often neglected by the consultant. They can provide individualized instruction to students, have access to reference materials to aid consultation efforts, and have insight into issues such as the teaching of reading, for example. At one elementary school, the consultant obtained materials from the librarian to aid a Level II consultation request from a teacher whose colleagues downstairs were complaining about the noise her students were making. This teacher encouraged physical exercise with her students as a means of letting off steam and building body stamina. Her students were jumping up and down doing calisthenics, and the floor was vibrating loudly. She asked the consultant for ideas on how to give the students this needed change of pace without disturbing other classes. The consultant, who was a psychologist with little knowledge of exercise or noise control, turned to the school librarian. The librarian found books on isometric exercises, which could be done quitely, and this material was passed on to the teacher. The consultant's role here was simply to act as a resource, which meant making use of the librarian. Because the librarian sees all the classes in the school, they may have a more global sense of what some of the common problems are, and thus can provide avenues for consultation entry.

Remedial or Basic Skills Teachers

Remedial or basic skills teachers provide remedial services under various forms of federal and other funding, otherwise known as Title I. They are often neglected by special services personnel because special education and tutorial programs are usually funded separately, and therefore are under separate bureaucracies. Yet these remedial teachers are experts in such fields as reading and math, and their skills need to be tapped. If reading is not being taught as effectively as it could be, the consultant could bring the remedial and regular teachers together for meetings and inservices on improving the teaching of reading. The consultant can share research, such as Carbo's (1987a, 1987b) findings that there is too much emphasis on phonics, and thereby try to change the emphasis of the reading curriculum. The impact on the school program is bound to be more global than it would be from efforts at consulting with one student or even one classroom teacher, and it may prevent referrals to special education.

At one elementary school, our special services team set as a goal for the school year the improvement of the teaching of reading. This goal reflected the reading difficulties faced by many students in the district and a districtwide needs assessment used by another department to schedule teacher inservices. The special services team brought in university experts on reading to summarize the research and discuss methodology (Levels III and IV interventions). The key guerrilla tactic, however, was to involve the basic skills teachers in planning the workshop. These teachers not only developed the outline and emphases, but functioned as a panel of discussants. At another workshop, they did demonstration teaching by videotape. Thus, they became models for other staff (rather than tutors to whom teachers referred students when they were not successful in teaching them to read).

Through this shared programming involvement, the team gained openings to consult with the basic skills classes, where they could have an impact on the teaching, tune in to the neediest students, and observe how they responded to expert teaching. This also had a preventive effect—helping students while they were still in these remedial classes, rather than waiting until they became special education students.

Teachers Grouped by Age and Experience

Teachers sometimes group themselves by age, especially younger teachers and those most experienced. Young teachers are often hungry for guidance and support and may welcome the consultant's interest. Sarason et al. (1966) cited what is often a serious neglect of new teachers by school administration. New teachers in our district, and I suspect in many others, get little in the way of supervision or support, although there has been a nationwide effort, in part fostered by the National Education Association, to improve teacher retention through mentoring programs. Despite this effort, first-year teachers in many schools "are woefully without the support that would allow them to move out of novice-like practice" (Sparks-Langer & Berstein Colton, 1991, p. 43). The importance of such support was illustrated in a study that showed that job satisfaction of special education teachers was closely related to the degree and nature of support from the principal or special education administrator (McManus & Kaufman, 1991).

When new teachers do not receive this attention, they tend to cluster together for mutual support. Such groupings can be entry points for the consultant. Sometimes consultants can help principals by supporting and encouraging the skills of new teachers in such areas as behavior management, lesson planning, and even research (Meyers's Level III). Support can start at simple levels. One special services staff member was helpful to a new teacher at an elementary school simply by finding remedial materials for her to use with students who had special needs. Technically, this was the principal's job, but he was too busy to provide that support. At a junior high school, a consultant helped a new teacher by reinforcing skills from an earlier inservice on "Assertive Discipline" (Canter, 1989).

One central issue here is building alliances, which is crucial to a consultant's successful functioning. Although new teachers are not the best allies in the short run, because they have little power or influence to make consultation entry happen, cultivating them will yield results as they gain influence. Conversely, the consultant needs to be wary of becoming associated with "deviant" staff people (Caplan, 1970). Some new teachers may be very aggressive and tend to pursue challenges to authority, causing difficulties for principals and administration. Although this is any staff member's prerogative, the consultant must be careful not to appear allied with an antiadministration position. However, such a situation is not typical, for, starting with the college professors who evaluate and grade their student teaching, new teachers tend to be trained to please and defer to authorities (Canning, 1991). The consultant can help encourage reflective thinking in new teachers.

A priority for effective entry into a school is to associate with those who have the existing power. Experienced teachers are the most valuable allies. They have a wealth of knowledge that many administrators neglect to tap. They know the pitfalls, what will and will not succeed in a school, and who can make things work. The consultant should get to know them, even though at first some may be resistant to consultation. Teachers are often expected to give and give, receiving little for their efforts, and therefore may be wary of the consultant's offer to help (Sarason, 1982).

They wonder what the catch is if they cooperate and tend to doubt that the consultant has any new wisdom to offer. Of course, the consultant does not have "wisdom" to impart per se. What he/she can offer is the skill in helping people come up with solutions—their solutions. Yes, the consultant may have some knowledge of educational research that teachers do not, but this is of little value unless teachers are motivated to ask about it. This motivation comes from Maslow's (1954) self-actualization need. Not all experienced teachers acknowledge the need to continue to grow in knowledge and skills. The consultant has to help them value themselves, recreating a basic acceptance of themselves as human beings and skilled professionals (Maslow's belongingness and esteem levels). By encouraging a sharing of their existing skills and ideas, the consultant may reawaken their need to share and then to grow.

Sarason (1982) notes that skeptical teachers sometimes appreciate it once the consultant actually puts in some time on their behalf. Experienced teachers can also be reached by tapping their need to guide younger staff. Using them as models, as in the example with the basic skills teachers, is a way of meeting their needs for recognition, and can help the consultant expand into more holistic consultation.

Power Brokers/Enablers

Another way of grouping teachers is according to their power (power brokers) or their ability to make things happen (enablers). It is incumbent upon the consultant to use guerrilla tactics to identify these key people and make them allies. The consultant must mingle with the teachers where he/she can observe them functioning; for example, eating regularly in the teachers' lunchroom is a good idea. An inside consultant, instead of always sitting with one group of friends, should move around to different tables each time he/she eats. It is useful to observe the seating patterns. Most teachers I have observed sit in the same place and with the same group each time they eat. Watch who leads the conversation at each table; who sits down first and who follows. Who sits with the principal or other staff leaders?

Also go to a teacher's meeting. Do the same lunchroom patterns follow? Who challenges administration? Are those people just noise makers or do they wield real power? Some of the real leaders are the quietest, but their position usually wins out at faculty meetings or when policies are written. Who are the negative resisters (staff who object to all proposals for change). Who gets chosen for special assignments? Who is picked to fill in for administrators in their absence? Who gets their way, has the run of the office, has the freedom to take time off, and so forth? Who has been doing the faculty developing and mentoring (Boice, 1989)? Faculty meetings are an ideal time to inform the power brokers and enablers of the consultants' different functions and to disabuse principals and teachers of their notion that the special service team is limited to testing children and removing troublesome ones from the classroom. The consultants' interaction with staff at these meetings can itself be a modeling of problem-solving behavior, as consultants use their skills to bring opposing power groups together and resolve conflicts.

Find out who are the union representatives. Often these people are strong and assertive, which may be the reason they were chosen by their colleagues to lead. Union people are often key "stake holders" in consultation projects, especially if the projects take up extra teacher time or change teacher roles (Rosenfield, 1992). An inside consultant should go to union meetings, get on a committee, and help the union with its projects. There are many union committee tasks that do not involve direct confrontation with administration (which the consultant would want to avoid). Such committees could range from those planning social events to those organizing continuing education. Both would be appropriate for the consultant's participation. It might not be appropriate for an outside consultant to go to union meetings, but certainly it would be in line to get to know the union leaders' concerns.

When the consultant is in the classroom often, some staff may raise the issue that the consultant is "supervising" the teacher (which is not permitted by administrators or union). This is particularly true when the consultant's method is instructional consultation (Rosenfield, 1987). In this method, the consultant examines how the teacher prepares instructional materials, how the lessons are organized, how student progress is evaluated, and so forth. Close union relationships can help eliminate union concerns about the consultant supervising union teachers, and provide an opportunity for union awareness of the consultant's role in facilitating staff development.

The union's own agenda should also be examined. What does the union want for its members? If one goal is professional growth and recognition, it is right in line with the consultant's goal. Both good consultants and unions want to see teacher empowerment, because empowerment is one of the best ways of tapping into teacher energy and creativity. Teacher creativity is often hidden under the need to defer to authority (Canning, 1991). Canning (1991) noted that such needs are learned in college, and her studies of new teachers showed that they had "lost touch with their voices" (p. 19) and instead tended to focus on what they felt they were supposed to say. Canning said that student teachers often want to be told what to do. When they suppress their own creativity, teachers are more likely to "dump" problems on consultants, because they lack the confidence and self-esteem to brainstorm their own solutions. Empowerment of teachers creates ownership of their problems. If teachers own more of the problems they face in the classroom, the consultant can more easily come in as an equal, rather than being cast into the role of the authority expert who will "save" the teacher.

Once the consultant identifies the power brokers, he/she should get to know them. This is not currying favor with power but recognizing the reality of dealing with the people with whom we must interact in order to make our program work. The consultant is seeking to help these people with their goals of advancing the status of their colleagues. Consultants do not have to agree with them all the time, but they should be aware of what these power brokers value, and the power brokers need to know that the consultant cares about what is important to them. Chances are that their agendas overlap with the consultant's. These may be professional agendas (such as improving the quality of schooling) or survival agendas (coping successfully with the state's or principal's evaluations). In some schools, the power brokers have more to say than the principal. They can sabotage or enable consultation efforts.

Counselors

The counselor, while considered a member of the special services staff for the purposes of this book, could also be considered a target for consultation entry by other consultants. Counselors, because of similarity in training, could be the closest ally of outside and inside consultants. Many counselors are also trained in consultation techniques, and the American Counseling Association, in Alexandria, Virginia, is a publisher of many school consultation materials.

Counselors are often referral sources for consultants, but they also tend to shift the more difficult cases to other special services personnel, such as social workers or psychologists, some of whom may have had more training in intensive counseling.

The guerrilla tactic here is to help counselors become more effective. Encouraging group counseling, perhaps with the consultant's help, is one way to reach more students. Such counseling, especially if it emphasizes wellness, can facilitate primary prevention (Commission on the Prevention of Mental–Emotional Disabilities, 1987; Freiberg, 1991). The Commission on the Prevention of Mental–Emotional Disabilities (1987) stated that alcoholism, auto accidents, abuse, prejudice, and unemployment are all factors that need early intervention. Using conflict management skills, structured groups could focus on dealing with parents, coping with depression or suicidal feelings, preventing involvement with drugs or alcohol, or handling aggressive behavior. The Commission noted the importance of schools working to develop competence in students to cope with life. This means handling aggression, solving social isolation, learning to cope with divorce, and so on. Integrity groups (Mowrer, 1972) can reinforce moral values such as honesty and self-disclosure. Groups can teach behavioral health and stress management along the lines of prevention noted by Thoresen and Eagleston (1985).

The consultant is in a position to encourage counselors to use consultation techniques to enhance their effectiveness with the teachers. If the consultant is a noncounselor, the counselor could also help the consultant. Many counselors are knowledgeable about consultation techniques and could be a good source of additional consultation skills. Many counselors know their students and staff well and can be valuable guides to the consultant. It can be beneficial to use counselors to help run inservice programs and to tap community resource people. The counselor, who is in the school daily, often functioning as the consultant's teammate, provides continuity to a consultation effort when teams and consultants are not in a given school every day. Counselors should be included in team meetings and become part of consultation intervention planning.

Once the consultant has considered points at which to enter to consult with teachers, he/she must look at the issue of what these teachers *need*.

TEACHER NEEDS

A Sense of Community

Teachers have strong social needs. After all, they often become teachers because of the need to work with others. In Maslow's (1954) hierarchy (discussed in earlier), such needs come under belongingness, a need to be valued by and become close emotionally to others. In the Holland (1966) scheme (see Chapter 5 for elaboration), the social theme is related to teachers' vocational interests. This personality theme emphasizes the need to work with and help others, and to work in groups of people, as opposed to working alone. Yet, in many schools the consultant finds teachers to be isolated. When they do meet as a group, it is for lectures and lists of procedures from administrators, and they have little chance to interact with their colleagues.

Sarason, in 1982, noted how isolated teachers are. Staff isolation was still an issue 7 years later when Boice (1989) made a strong case for psychologists to act as faculty "developers" to reduce staff isolation by encouraging collegial communication. He pushed for faculty participation in the planning of programs to help teachers develop, and Giammatteo and Giammatteo (1981) suggested that teachers be supervised in groups to encourage sharing of personal goals and values. Such programs can meet a variety of needs as long as they bring staff together. Such approaches could include physical fitness, which, although not immediately relevant to school programming, has a strong social component. Physical fitness also works as a stress reducer and, in the long run, could reduce absences from illness.

Attendance concerns are one incentive to convince administrators to run such programs, and the consultant could find the right people to set it up.

A teacher support group is another means of improving a sense of community. Gersch and Rawkins (1987) used video recordings in such groups to develop a behavioral treatment approach with children who had severe learning disabilities. I have used groups in elementary and junior high school settings to help disenfranchised, isolated teachers support each other and develop coping methods to deal with students and administration. It is difficult to find times when all target teachers are available, but the effort is worthwhile. Teachers in such groups reported less isolation and more of a sense of belonging and efficacy.

Bringing together special education and regular education teachers can accomplish social goals as well. Graden (1989) stressed the importance of such collaboration. Friend and Bauwens (1988) suggested that learning disability teachers could consult with regular education teachers as a means of reducing professional barriers and providing a greater sense of community (and ability to cope with difficult students). (Such consultation has been going on for a long time but not in every school district.) McManus and Kaufman (1991) found that few teachers of self-contained classes sought help from regular education teachers. At schools in which I have worked, this is also true at both the elementary and secondary levels. There is also no reason why regular education teachers could not initiate consultations with special education teachers. Nevertheless, despite isolated exceptions—as in the Knight et al. (1981) study—one rarely finds mutual support by regular and special education staff at the typical school.

The regular education initiative (Hallahan et al., 1988) places special education students in regular classes and modifies the teaching in those classes to meet the needs of the students with special needs. Here the skills of the classroom teacher can be improved with consultation, which brings teachers together as allies. Staff community occurs when the specialist teacher comes into the regular classroom to help (or vice versa).

The Vermont Consulting Teacher Program (Knight et al., 1981) was one of the first to place resource room specialists in the regular classroom to help students with learning problems. They did so with the cooperation of university faculty consultants and field-based consulting teachers in public schools. Since then, many other programs have been developed. Boles and Truen (1992) developed university contacts so that teacher interns could free up staff to do team teaching and provide more support in the regular classroom for special needs students who previously had to be pulled out of the class for special instruction.

Professional Growth

Bardon and Bennett (1974) noted how important it was for the special services team member to improve teacher performance. Consultants must help to further teachers' growth. Blum, Butler, and Olson (1987) suggested "vision building," essentially, a leadership program that pushed for excellence, in which staff were helped to focus on their own priorities and goals. Consultation that respects each teacher's own "style" (Conoley & Conoley, 1988) also can create an openness for growth. A flexible, democratic teacher may be more open to consultation about issues of teacher attitudes, while a more structured, rigid teacher might prefer to work on improvement around curricular issues.

Saporito and Ross (1987), in defining the consultant's role, emphasized the importance of working with administration to define or redefine the organization's philosophy in the hopes of developing more strategic plans. Such long-term plans anticipate the skills that staff must develop to meet future demands. An organization also needs to have purpose, for without purpose, professional growth cannot be directed. Consultants can help teachers articulate how they want to grow, and identify their resources (their own and from other staff) to facilitate such growth.

Idol and West (1987) addressed this issue, studying eight programs. These programs utilized special education teachers to work with regular education staff. The special educators were taught how to consult, using process skills of communication such as active listening, support of others, conflict resolution, negotiation, paraphrasing, constructive use of feelings, and so on (see Appendix A).

Consultants were trained in data-based instruction, applied behavior analysis, instructional design, curriculum and technology, systems development, and change (all in the Vermont studies) as well as in services to special needs learners, program development, management and evaluation, referral systems, curriculum-based assessment, literature on effective teaching, data collection, collaboration, and resource identification, among other skills (Idol & West, 1987, pp. 477–479).

Idol and West maintain that even such thorough training is not enough. Criteria must be developed to check whether the process and knowledge skills, as well as the *outcomes*, are successful. Process criteria measure how well a person is able to reflect back another person's thoughts or statements, or to tune in to hidden meanings. Knowledge criteria are simply measures of a person's knowledge, about such things as what teaching techniques have been shown to be the most effective, or what special needs a retarded student has. Outcome criteria measure success in consultation training, and could include logbooks on the use of communication skills or written analyses of a systems problem or a plan for monitoring service delivery. Measuring outcomes of consultation training includes looking at actual products (i.e., written or behavioral results) to see whether the student consultant's skills have improved. Products also include training plans, practicum projects (what the consultant trainee will actually carry out for practice), or trainees' case studies. It is perhaps even more important that the consultant develop criteria that actually specify changes in consultee *behavior* as a result of consultation efforts. Although Idol and West studied projects as late as 1986, only the University of Vermont project actually developed plans of action for bringing about growth in classroom teachers (the consultees) (see also Bergan, 1985; Bergan & Kratochwill, 1990). Training that stimulates teachers professional growth requires that the knowledge and skills imparted be proven to effectively change others.

Another way for teachers to grow is to become involved in research (Casanova, 1989). The consultant can present research data on concerns that they raise. Their role in the analysis of ideas will encourage collegiality as well as research production. Casanova notes that teachers rarely get to do this kind of philosophical reflection, which can have a positive effect on professional growth and staff productivity. At one of our junior high schools, the special services team involved the discipline staff in simple research to identify referral patterns and types of infractions. The team and disciplinarians reviewed the records of suspended students and the list of referring teachers. A frequency chart was developed to tally the referral patterns from different staff members and by type of infraction. The discipline staff indicated their priorities regarding which infractions they wanted to address, and a group of students was identified for a group counseling approach. The disciplinary teachers' participation in the initial research made them more cooperative with the consultant later. This was in part because their concerns were valued, but also because of personal growth, as they were able to see for themselves the value of participating in research.

Would-be consultants must be aware that the resistance of school staff to extensive research procedures is "legendary" (Rosenfield, 1987). If the consultant attempts to stimulate teachers to do research, it should be simple and not take up too much of the time resources that teachers must allocate.

Boles and Truen (1992) solved this time dilemma by convincing administration to restructure the master school schedule to give all teachers time to meet and plan. By bringing in full-time teacher interns for training, regular teachers were freed to do research of their own design. Teachers were encouraged (by their peers) to take time to research problems of interest to them as a means of staff development. For example, while one intern taught a writing lesson, the teacher conducted interviews and observed strategies that differentiated good writers from others. She wanted to find better ways to teach writing and was able to pursue this goal because of the schedule restructuring which freed her up to do planning.

Efficacy

"Efficacy" means the power to produce effects or results. Teachers need to feel that they are not pawns in a large system (Sergiovanni & Starratt, 1988) where change is beyond their control. They need to be respected for their intellect and to feel they can contribute to the improvement of the system. When they are treated like children (Ashton & Webb, 1986), when their drawers and files are checked for cleanliness by the principal before permitting them to leave for the summer, the message is: "You are children, who cannot be responsible." Such an attitude makes teachers defiant and/or lowers their self-esteem. Moreover, this approach stifles a teacher's sense of being able to cope with the environment or have an impact on the school.

Professionals need to have influence. The consultant must be sensitive to how those needs can be met. The consultant's role here is to help with such empowerment by interceding with administration to establish a greater role for staff in policy, planning, and procedures (Harvey, 1989). Conducting an inservice on stress (discussed later in this chapter) is an example of how such intervention can be accomplished. The consultant also needs to support teachers as "executives" in their own classroom (Shore & Vieland, 1989) by helping them maintain control. As such, the consultant becomes an "enabler" (Trachtman, 1981), helping teachers and students interact more effectively.

Teacher efficacy is based on beliefs that students can learn and that teachers can be effective (Armor et al., cited in Sergiovanni & Starratt, 1988). Ashton and Webb (1986) demonstrated that teachers who feel effective have a positive impact on student behavior and achievement. Conoley and Conoley (1988) cite Schein's earlier work in industry to improve problem-solving skills via group approaches. Here the consultant plays a big part in building on teacher efficacy by enhancing teacher skills and confidence, pride, professionality, innovativeness (Sarason et al., 1966), and self-esteem. In turn, when they see that their efforts are being encouraged and praised, teachers take more responsibility for what they do. The consultant can further this process by helping principals support and praise steps that teachers take to become more efficacious and helping them create opportunities for teachers to have more of an impact.

The consultant is more likely to gain teacher cooperation with interventions that the teacher can implement directly (Martens, Witt, Elliott, & Darveaux, 1985) and that require small or moderate amounts of time. Teacher control over the intervention and the time to exert that control are crucial to enhancing efficacy. Although teachers prefer the collaborative approach (Pryzwansky & White, 1983), Erchul and Chewning (1990) found in actual verbal analyses of consultation sessions that consultants *controlled* the consultation (when using Bergan's behavioral consultation) and consultees tended to be passive, accepting, and cooperative. In later stages of consultation, however, the consultees took more control of the sessions.

The issue here may be teacher perception of control rather than what actually happened in the verbal transcript. It is also possible that the behavioral approach, because of its highly scientific nature, may require more directiveness on the part of the consultant than do more collaborative approaches. Nevertheless, the importance of analyzing actual transcripts of consultation, using the techniques of Kratochwill and Bergan (1990) and Erchul and Chewning (1990), cannot be underestimated if the degree of the consultant's, and the teacher's, professional growth is to be evaluated.

The consultant's efforts to find programs already in the school (Collins, Brash, Watkin, Venhorst, & Connolly, 1988) that could be utilized by teachers facing problems can help teachers feel more effective, as well as reduce special education referrals. After all, efficacy also means knowing the resources; knowing what to do to find answers. The consultation report (as shown in Chapter 3, Figure 3.1) initially seems to be a way simply to write what happened at a consultation meeting. However, the options that are listed on the form serve to jog teachers' minds about alternatives to special education placement. When the alternatives are in writing, they become harder to ignore in a discussion of options.

Performance Investment

Documenting Results

Performance investment refers to the degree of involvement and enthusiasm teachers develop for their work and for the consultation interventions. For teachers to feel a performance investment, they must see that benefits will accrue to them from consultation projects. Friend and Bauwens (1988) recommend that the consultant gather data on the effectiveness of consultation so that teachers can see that it is working. In behavioral consultation, Bergan (1985), Kratochwill and Van Someren (1985), and Kratochwill and Bergan (1990) actually record the verbalizations between consultant and consultee to determine the effectiveness of the consultation. Grimes (1981) urged consultants to write a memo to the teacher after each consultation, summarizing the data discussed. Our teams use a department form, the Consultation Progress Report (see Chapter 3, Figure 3.2). This is filled out jointly by consultant and teacher and lists the responsibilities for the consultation and the data used to check those responsibilities. This method accounts for the time spent in consultation (Roth, 1980) and is important because teachers and consultants are always held accountable for their time. It results in a clear description of how the consultation has worked, and can encourage teachers about the progress they or their students are making. It takes courage to use such forms, as failures also become more evident. But evaluation of consultations is necessary, and to be effective, special services personnel must face failed results and find ways to improve approaches.

Measuring Satisfaction

Another approach to a more general evaluation of the consultant's efforts could be a general satisfaction survey. Such a survey gives teachers another means of voicing their feelings about what is happening in consultation. One that our child study team developed (Figure 4.1) uses ratings on a 5-point scale as well as open-ended questions, so that teachers can express themselves freely. We gave this form to every teacher involved with the child study team, whether we did traditional evaluation or consultation. A similar form was used for administrators (see Chapter 2, Figure 2.1). By and large, the results were favorable, but a number of negative comments indicated that the teachers felt free to be honest. Most of the negatives dealt with insufficient speed of response to referrals.

Erchul and Chewning's (1990) Consultant Evaluation Form (Figure 4.2), a refinement of Gallesich and Derby's (1976) Consultant Assessment Form, focuses more specifically on consultation than does our form (which is oriented more to the totality of special services team practice). Gallesich (1982) developed an expanded form, the Consultation Evaluation Survey (Figure 4.3).

CONSULTATION TEAM
CHILD STUDY TEAM RATING FORM FOR TEACHERS
This year you referred at least one student to the child study team. Please
answer these brief questions to help us evaluate and improve our services.

	Very dissatisfied				Very satisfied

I. Rate your satisfaction with:
   A. The time it took for the child study
       team to first respond to your
       consultation request — 1 2 3 4 5
   B. The usefulness of the consultation
       meetings — 1 2 3 4 5
   C. How fast the student was evaluated
       (if evaluation was recommended) — 1 2 3 4 5
   D. The ongoing support from, and
       communication with child study team — 1 2 3 4 5

II. Rate your satisfaction with these other child
    study team services and functions:
   A. Quality of inservice training sessions
      run by the child study team — 1 2 3 4 5
   B. The child study team's professionalism — 1 2 3 4 5
   C. The child study team's role in helping to
      improve communication between staff
      and administrators — 1 2 3 4 5
   D. The child study team's efforts to impact
      on school programming — 1 2 3 4 5

III. Comments about our child study team's work:

_____

_____

IV. The best thing about our child study team is:

_____

_____

V. The worst thing about our child study team is:

_____

_____

School: _____

Position or title: _____

Date: _____

Name: _____

(Not Required)

FIGURE 4.1. Form for teacher's evaluation of child study team. Permission
to reproduce this form is granted to purchasers of *Entry Strategies for School
Consultation* for professional use with their clients.

1. The consultant was generally helpful.
2. The consultant offered useful information.
3. The consultant's ideas as to the primary goals of schools were similar to my own ideas.
4. The consultant helped me find alternative solutions to problems.
5. The consultant was a good listener.
6. The consultant helped me identify useful resources.
7. The consultant fit well into the school's environment.
8. The consultant encouraged me to consider a number of points of view.
9. The consultant viewed his or her role as a collaborator rather than as an expert.
10. The consultant helped me find ways to apply the content of our discussions to specific pupil or classroom situations.
11. The consultant was able to offer assistance without completely "taking over" the management of problems.
12. I would request services from this consultant again, assuming that other consultants were available.

FIGURE 4.2. The Consultant Evaluation Form. The consultee circles the number of each applicable item after a consultation session is held. From Erchul and Chewning (1990, p. 9). Copyright 1990 by William P. Erchul. Reprinted by permission.

These forms can help teachers look at the product of their efforts and evaluate it. The consultant's openness represents the kind of collaborative approach that Pryzwansky and White (1983) state teachers overwhelmingly favor. A collaborative approach encourages teacher control (Hamway & Elias, 1988), especially if the approach fits the teacher's own conceptualization (Johnson et al., 1988). Performance investment, then, is created when the consultant can prove that teachers benefit from their efforts to improve.

Utilizing Data

The consultant can aid teacher efforts to improve by gathering important student and classroom data and teaching consultees to make sense of it. Joel Meyers (n.d.) noted that when test and classroom observation data are gathered but *not* used as a basis for consultation with teachers, students end up being referred to and evaluated by the special services team for special education placement (instead of teachers taking on the responsibility for solutions). Often this results in the ownership of the referral problem being switched from the teacher to the team. Psychological, social case history, speech, and educational evaluations, done as part of the consulting or referral

CONSULTATION EVALUATION SURVEY

Your organization_____Date_____
Consultant's name_____
Number of years you have worked in this type of organization_____
Sex (circle one)   Male   Female
Have you had previous experience with consultants?
Yes   No
To what extent have you made use of the consultant this year?
___ Not at all
___ Very little, 1 or 2 times
___ To a moderate extent, about 3 to 6 times
___ To a considerable extent, about 6 to 10 times
___ To a great extent, more than 10 times
In general, how helpful has the consultant been to you? (Circle the number that
is most descriptive)
     Not at all 1 2 3 4 5 6 7   Very helpful
Did you work with the consultant in a group situation?
Yes   No
Did you work with the consultant on an individual basis?
Yes   No

Please respond to the following items by circling the number that best describes
your perception of your consultant. response options range from 1 (not at all
descriptive) to 7 (very descriptive). If an item does not seem applicable to your
consultant, circle N.A.

The consultant:
  1. Offers useful information.   1 2 3 4 5 6 7 N.A.
  2. Understands my working environment.   1 2 3 4 5 6 7 N.A.
  3. Presses his/her ideas and solutions.   1 2 3 4 5 6 7 N.A.
  4. Is skilled in forming good working.
     relationships.   1 2 3 4 5 6 7 N.A.
  5. Is a good listener.   1 2 3 4 5 6 7 N.A.
  6. Helps me find alternative solutions to problems.   1 2 3 4 5 6 7 N.A.
  7. Increases my self-confidence.   1 2 3 4 5 6 7 N.A.
  8. Helps me identify resources to use in
     problem solving.   1 2 3 4 5 6 7 N.A.
  9. Is not concerned with my point of view.   1 2 3 4 5 6 7 N.A.
 10. Encourages me to make my own decisions.   1 2 3 4 5 6 7 N.A.
 11. Helps me find ways to apply content of
     our discussions to specific situations.   1 2 3 4 5 6 7 N.A.
 12. Respects values that are different from
     his/hers.   1 2 3 4 5 6 7 N.A.
 13. Fits easily into our work setting.   1 2 3 4 5 6 7 N.A.
 14. Stimulates me to see situations in more
     complex ways.   1 2 3 4 5 6 7 N.A.
 15. Relies on one approach to solving
     problems.   1 2 3 4 5 6 7 N.A.
 16. Explains his/her ideas clearly.
 17. Has difficulty understanding my concerns.   1 2 3 4 5 6 7 N.A.

18. Encourages me to try a variety of
    interventions.   1 2 3 4 5 6 7 N.A.
19. Helps me in ways consistent with my
    own needs.   1 2 3 4 5 6 7 N.A.
20. Encourages communication between me
    and others with whom I work.   1 2 3 4 5 6 7 N.A.
21. Increases my understanding of basic
    psychological principles.   1 2 3 4 5 6 7 N.A.
22. Makes helpful suggestions.   1 2 3 4 5 6 7 N.A.
23. Does not appreciate the pressures of my job.   1 2 3 4 5 6 7 N.A.
24. Makes me feel comfortable in discussing
    sensitive problems.   1 2 3 4 5 6 7 N.A.
25. Encourages our work group to cooperate.   1 2 3 4 5 6 7 N.A.
26. Supports my efforts to solve problems.   1 2 3 4 5 6 7 N.A.
27. Has knowledge relevant to my work.   1 2 3 4 5 6 7 N.A.
28 Helps me understand myself better.   1 2 3 4 5 6 7 N.A.
29. Helps me develop a wider range of problem-
    solving skills.   1 2 3 4 5 6 7 N.A.
30. Rushes into premature solutions.   1 2 3 4 5 6 7 N.A.
31. Is sensitive to my feelings.   1 2 3 4 5 6 7 N.A.
32. Helps me to see my situation more objectively.   1 2 3 4 5 6 7 N.A.
33. Knows when and how to ask good questions.   1 2 3 4 5 6 7 N.A.
34. Is reliable about appointments.   1 2 3 4 5 6 7 N.A.

This consultant will not be consulting in the future. What suggestions do you
have to help him/her improve in consultation skills? Remember, this information
will NOT be used for grading: it will be extremely helpful to your consultant as
feedback.

What did you like most about his/her work?
What did you like least about his/her work?
If you did not use this consultant, why not?

FIGURE 4.3. Consultation Evaluation Survey. From Gallesich (1982, p. 59).
Copyright 1982 by Jossey Bass, Inc. Reprinted by permission.

process, need to be shared with the teacher in such a manner as to
make them useful in intervention *before* considering classification
under special education and/or other placements. Such data can be
recorded on the Consultation Progress Report (Figure 3.2). Such
sharing is an entry strategy, because it starts a dialogue between
consultant and teacher.

Teaching recommendation garnered from such tests as a Wechsler
Intelligence Scale for Children—Revised (WISC-R) or WISC-III
(Third Edition) need to be spelled out in a practical way that teachers
can use. The WISC-III Compilation (Whitworth & Sutton, 1993) is
a good example of how test results on each subtest can be translated

into practical lessons in the classroom. This guide provides specific course objectives as well as teaching materials for WISC areas in which a student is weak. Similar course objectives, educational recommendations, and strategies are also available on computer interpretations of such tests as the WISC-R or WISC-III, Wechsler Adult Intelligence Scale—Revised (WAIS-R), Stanford–Binet IV, and Woodcock–Johnson Achievement Test—Revised, on programs such as Report Writer (product of Psychological Assessment Resources, Odessa, Florida). Of course, published recommendations for interventions are no guarantee of success, but they give the teacher and consultant an opportunity to make some use of the test data and raise hypotheses that can be tested.

Piersal (cited in Bergan, 1985) felt that traditional assessment could easily lead into problem-solving behavioral consultation in the classroom to help assess the environment there as it relates to the student's areas of weakness on these tests. Test results that indicate strengths and deficits could also lead to classroom instructional consultation using Gagne's (1977) learning hierarchies as a means of assessing where the student is (Rosenfield, 1987) on the path to development of sequential skills.

Our Consultation Progress Report (see Chapter 3, Figure 3.2) can be used to record this kind of data, as well as the results of the intervention. It is only by evaluating intervention results that recommendations from testing or other observational data can really be tested. For example, if the intelligence testing suggests that a visual approach would be helpful in teaching reading, the consultant would test this hypothesis by first obtaining baseline data on reading rate or accuracy. One could use a curriculum-based assessment that measures the number of correct words a student reads orally per minute (CWPM). These data would be analyzed to decide if and where improvement would be required. A student reading at 15 CWPM might have improving to 32 CWPM as an objective. The intervention could be a visual approach to teach the words, perhaps a flash card, Rebus, or tachistoscopic method, all of which deemphasize phonetic factors. Progress would then be measured by the increase in CWPM. Reversion to the regular method of teaching reading would be a further test of whether the visual method was better. Continued measurement of CWPM at different intervals would have to be done and, ideally, the visual method again reinstated.

Teachers who learn to utilize assessments and teaching methods that are meaningful to classroom change and confirm their efforts through effective evaluation should increase their performance investment. Change in the consultee could also be considered a criterion of consultation effectiveness in increasing performance investment (Bardon, 1985). Bardon suggests studying consultee behavior, attitudes, feelings, and intentions, if we are to understand how effective our consulting efforts are.

Encouraging Teamwork

The consultant can also increase performance investment by encouraging staff to become involved in team teaching (Friend & Bauwens, 1988) (Meyers's Levels III and IV). In such teaching, one teacher teams with another to lend a skill the latter does not have, or to enhance the curriculum by sharing knowledge. This kind of opportunity to contribute to and benefit from colleagues' knowledge and support can encourage people to question standard procedures, experiment with curriculum variations, monitor themselves, and grow. Teachers need backing from peers, but they rarely experience it without teacher groups or teams at their school.

In view of the above, it is clear that in order to achieve successful entry with teachers, the consultant also must become comfortable working with *groups*. One way to further understand groups is to look at different types of group functioning.

There are "work" groups and "psychological" groups. Work groups have specific tasks to accomplish. Psychological groups are those that meet the members' mutual needs and share common goals. The focus in this discussion will be on faculty work groups to enhance staff effectiveness. Because a group is designated as a work group, that does not mean that it is effective as a psychological group. Rather, it may have been organized to maintain the status quo or the regularities of the school (Sarason, 1982). An example might be a curriculum committee or faculty senate with no real power to make substantive changes. A psychological group is not necessarily an effective work group either. An effective group (Likert, 1961) is one in which members help each individual to achieve his/her potential, link goals harmoniously, and create a sense of mutual confidence and trust without losing task focus.

Examining Group Functioning

One can evaluate how a faculty group functions using Reddin's Team Analysis Key, part of his Team Style Diagnostic Test (cited in Sergiovanni & Starratt, 1988; Reddin, 1994). This key uses eight dimensions of faculty group effectiveness:

1. Enthusiasm and commitment for group goals and purposes
2. Quantity and quality of member contributions to the group
3. Quality of listening by members one to another
4. Creativity exhibited in problem solving
5. Ways the group handles conflict and disagreements
6. Quality and nature of leadership
7. Methods and means of making decisions
8. Ways the group evaluates its performance

And eight descriptors applied to these dimensions of group behavior on any *one* occasion:

A. Little interest in getting the job done
B. More interest in group harmony than accomplishment
C. More interest in argument than accomplishment
D. Little consistent focus on the problem
E. Much attention to following procedure and established patterns
F. Much attention to development of a team
G. Clear-cut attempt to stay with the problem
H. Enthusiastic team attempt to look at the problem as broadly and deeply as possible.

For each dimension, three of these eight descriptors are chosen as most applicable to how the group functions in that area. The three are rated on a scale of 1–10 in terms of how closely each describes the group. One might rate a group on dimension 1 (enthusiasm and commitment) by choosing descriptors A, E, and F (interest, following procedure, and team development) as most applicable. The ratings for the 3 descriptors must add up to 10, but can be apportioned according to how much weight the observer wants to give each. If for dimension 1 the consultant gave ratings of 4, 5, and 1 (A, E, and F), the consultant felt the group lacked interest in getting the job done (A), focused excessively on procedure (E), and made only minor efforts at team development (F). Once all the dimensions have been given three ratings each, the ratings are added for each descriptor, to see which best applies to the group (the one with the most points).

A group scoring high on descriptor A (little interest in getting a job done, for example, is a group in flight, with a leader who Reddin (cited in Sergiovanni & Starratt, 1988) describes as a "deserter." The members display little energy toward task completion. Conflict is minimized and creativity is low. Leadership may be absent, and there are rarely attempts to improve group performance.

Groups scoring high on descriptor E, on the other hand, do get their work done, but in a formal manner with very defined procedures guiding members' contributions. The group evaluates itself in a functional manner, but often by comparing itself to other groups. The group has a functional leader, unlike in the previous example, but one who functions in a bureaucratic manner (Sergiovanni & Starratt, 1988). The complete list of groups categorized by Reddin are:

If the group rates high on descriptor:	The group is:	The group's leader could be described as:
A	In flight	Deserter
B	Dependent	Missionary
C	Fighting	Autocrat
D	Mixed	Compromiser
E	Procedural	Bureaucrat
F	Creative	Developer
G	Productive	Benevolent autocrat
H	Problem-solving	Executive

The "dependent" group is more interested in maintaining harmony, and so production is sacrificed so as to avoid conflict. The "missionary" leader keeps everyone agreeing but is also weak. The better functioning groups are the "creative," "productive," and "problem-solving" ones, which focus respectively on member self-development (F), high task orientation (G), and deep examination of problems coupled with high task orientation (H).

Look at the school where you work, see if you recognize any of these groups and leaders, and evaluate your own approach to working with groups. Try the Reddin Team Analysis (Reddin, 1994) the next time you go to a faculty committee meeting. (It can be obtained from W. J. Reddin and Associates, P. O. Box 324, Fredericton, N. B., E3B 4Y9, Canada.)

Becoming a Group Leader

The consultant who is handling the group needs to have a sense of what common threads run through the discussions and what the opposing views are, and then help the group find common ground. The consultant's goal in Reddin's scheme, ultimately, is to help teachers (or him/herself) become "executives," but productive roles can also be as "developers" and "benevolent autocrats."

My own experience suggests that the consultant should create respect for differences and individuality by not taking sides, by using mediation, and by trying to restate what each person is saying. The leader should have opposing sides restate what they heard their opponents say. Keep the group *task*-focused rather than *blame*-focused. It is possible for the consultant to provide support even if he/she is not the leader. Consultants should help summarize what has been said at different points, encourage frank communication, and create an atmosphere where people can say what they feel without fear of criticism.

When the consultant helps create an effective group, he/she will find that the group is characterized by a high motivation to *influence,* as well as to accept the environment (Likert, 1961). The consultant, then, must create enthusiasm, which is tempered by acceptance. The consultant's ability to focus on groups in these ways is important in achieving entry with teachers. The consultant needs to serve such work groups, help them accomplish tasks, and encourage good group problem solving. Teachers' investment in their own job performance will no doubt be enhanced if they feel the groups in which they work are functional and effective.

Being available to serve teacher groups is an entry strategy, whereas actually working in them is a consultation intervention. However, there is overlap here, because good intervention in such groups leads to further entry opportunities to expand into holistic consultation, especially if the group begins to have the influence that Likert implies can occur. Intervening to empower teachers increases the consultant's impact on the larger school system. For more on groups and team functioning, see Chapter 3.

Smooth Relationships with Administrators

The special services staff or consultant smoothes the way for teachers to reach administrators and vice versa. One way to do this is to clarify misconceptions about the consultant's role. At one school, I was asked to work with a poorly functioning teacher, ostensibly to gather data so the teacher could be fired. At least this was the teacher's conception of the principal's agenda and the consultant's role. I took pains to clarify with the teacher that my role was to facilitate professional growth (a Level III intervention), a role that precluded aiding and abetting any administrative disciplinary action. I could prove this only by working on the teacher's priorities and allowing her to control the problem identification and goal setting processes. The teacher was able to improve once she realized that my goals were purely to help her set her own directions for improvement in teaching skills. More important, the communication between the teacher and principal improved, as she realized that I was not the principal's tool but had been brought in with sincere motivations on the part of administration. The principal, in understanding the consultation process and the steps being taken in the classroom, began to see this teacher's strengths and increased the level of support for the teacher.

Entry with teachers involves creating supports from administration to make the teacher's job easier, which are Level IV interventions. One way to do this is for the consultant to facilitate more flexible class groupings (Wrenn, 1967; Reger, cited in Magary, 1967). At one elementary school, the consultant was able to find a loophole in the regulations to make special education tutoring available to unclassified students. Opening up resources this way (a Level IV intervention) involved negotiations with administration and was seen as another source of support by teachers.

The consultant should try to open up the school for new activities and programs. The aforementioned training of junior high school students to orient incoming seventh graders is one example. In another effort, the consultants tried to create a self-contained seventh grade—a new program to meet provide the structure that students entering a large junior high school for the first time require. Although this effort was unsuccessful, self-contained seventh grade classes did develop later at other junior high schools. This kind of networking often takes place when consultants attempt to establish programs, so that, even if the consultant fails, it stimulates thought in others who may later have the power to develop such programs.

Time Investment

Meyers's work on adapting Caplan's (1970) levels of consultation to school settings gives the consultant options of where to intervene. The use of any such conceptualization requires an investment of time. The consultant must limit interventions to those on which he/she effectively can follow through (Grubb, 1981) and must give the teachers enough time so that many students can be reached.

Teachers need to know how to utilize consultation if it is to be beneficial. Training must be practical and experiential, not just didactic. Good consultation training, whether for the consultant or for the teacher, requires direct observation, self-monitoring, role play, modeling, reinforcement, and feedback (Kratochwill & Van Someren, 1985). West, Idol, and Cannon (1987) emphasize guided practice as well. All of these are superior to the typical inservice program of

1 ½ to 3 hours in which the special services person or consultant explains his/her role or in which methods are discussed. Teachers need to experience what consultation is like, and only their direct involvement in it makes training meaningful. The consultant's communication at such inservices needs to be empathic and genuine but also characterized by an honest persuasiveness (not coercion) (Parsons & Meyers, 1984).

How does the consultant create readiness for such intensive training? Training must start early, at the university level, as advocated by Parsons and Meyers (1984) and Idol and West (1987). As a special services staff member in the schools, the consultant does not control that. However, there are things that the consultant can do. One of our special services team members arranged to orient student teachers to the role of the special services team, and in doing so prepared them for the scrutiny and openness required for involvement in scientific consulting approaches. Consultants should take advantage of this opportunity to publicize their consultant role and prepare young people for the benefits of self-scrutiny and the challenges of this personal stretching process. Do not hesitate to involve student teachers in modeling and practice, as noted above, if their internship supervisor approves.

Fewer Burdens

The more people the consultant can influence, the greater the power of the consultation. Part of the consultant's task is to demonstrate to teachers, while doing his/her work, that the administration, as well as the teachers, is responsible for change. If teachers see an effort to reduce their burdens, they are less likely to see the consultant as an agent of the administration.

For example, teachers faced with student disruption are much more likely to pitch in on a task if they see administration taking action on their recommendations. In one of our elementary schools, where students were disruptive when going from class to the lunchroom, the special services team tapped the teachers' ideas of what to do. Many of their suggestions were related to Meyers's Level IV interventions (i.e., they had to do more with school rules and policies than with techniques of *their* managing of the students; Level II). The consultant relayed these ideas to the principal, and suggested that the necessary solutions were primarily to be found at a programmatic level (e.g., in lunch dismissal times and clear places for the students to line up) rather than with the teachers.

Some principals might have assumed that the teachers were inept at handling their classes. Our consultant's approach prevented the principal from criticizing teachers for the poor behavior of the classes. Certainly the teachers felt there were additional steps *they* could take to improve the situation, and they did not resent having to do them because (1) some of the other solutions came from their brainstorming and (2) the consultant involved administration in helping them. The consultant's efforts were aimed at easing teacher burdens while helping them to develop solutions.

Holding inservice training presents an opportunity to impact on teacher burdens as well. Our special services team prevailed on a principal to permit a needs assessment of teacher concerns prior to running a stress workshop for them. The idea was based on studies (National Institute for Occupational Safety and Health, 1987) showing that traditional stress management programs for teachers (relaxation, assertion, etc.) had only temporary value, and that the major stresses facing teachers were *ongoing* and a function of school *policies* and procedures.

The teachers in this elementary school identified a lack of substitute teachers, and resultant dumping of the absent teachers' students in their classes, as a major source of daily stress. The principal agreed to have the special services team do a workshop addressing these issues, as he too was stressed by the problem of obtaining substitutes. The workshop was well received, because the teachers felt it responded to their needs. While individual stress management techniques were also taught, methods for changing school and district approaches to this problem were emphasized, and the principal was given important data from the workshop's problem-solving groups. This workshop played an important part in the ultimate resolution by the district of these difficulties, which was another way of easing burdens on teachers. This type of intervention represented moving from a Level III approach to teacher stress to a Level IV intervention with the system.

Such sessions also serve to expand teachers' perceptions of the consultant's role, and help administration view the consultant as someone who can provide solutions. These solutions, rather than coming from the (incorrectly perceived) consultant as all-knowing expert, instead come from a reenergized, empowered school staff, for which the consultant has become a catalyst. Such an approach can also begin to remediate the above-noted passivity that some teachers have (Keys, 1983).

Because few school administrators tune into teacher pressures, other than for evaluation purposes (Caplan, 1970; Sarason, 1982), the consultant has a real opportunity. Consultants can teach techniques of observation, reinforcement, communication skills, and the like, but their concern for the personal pressures teachers undergo can provide real support and create allies as well. This does not mean that the consultant *treats* the teacher (see Caplan, 1970), but his/her ability to use listening skills and empathy (see Appendix A, on communication skills) may provide openings for teachers to seek solutions to their lack of classroom effectiveness due to personal pressures.

Some teachers need to be referred for psychotherapy, and being a psychotherapist is not the role of the consultant. Some teachers need career counseling to find a more satisfying or less stressful field, better suited to their abilities. The consultant can make such referrals, and this is often a more acceptable means of moving a poor teacher out of the field (rather than administrative censure or firing). If the consultant can become a trusted person, such teachers will open up to him/her and appreciate being steered in other directions, because they probably have had such thoughts themselves, and are likely to be under much stress, having made a poor vocational choice.

When the consultant models or helps the teacher think through a better approach, and the teacher is able to follow through with results, the burdens of a difficult class or student who is not learning are immediately eased. This occurred in a junior high school class when I modeled group counseling in the classroom. Teachers began to see alternative ways to handle the outbursts of difficult students. Such modeling also occurred when our learning consultant demonstrated techniques for increasing spoken language in an elementary school classroom. Teachers fearful of classes getting out of hand if they gave inner-city students an increased opportunity to verbalize, began to find their classes more enjoyable, and their relationships with students improved because of the improved frequency of verbal discussion.

Much of the research on effective education (some of which goes back many years) supports the notion of encouraging teachers to foster verbally active classes where students stimulate them with questions (Liddle, cited in Magary, 1967; Rutter et al., 1979; Sarason, 1982). Yet even now, in the 1990s, I have seen too many classes where lecture and seat work are instead the norm.

SUMMARY

Effective entry to consult with teachers requires knowledge of the school culture and climate, which I have described here and related to methods of entry. Effective entry also requires knowing with which groups to intervene, and I have discussed some of the major teacher groupings with which to explore entry. Knowledge of culture and climate also implies an awareness of teachers' needs, for community, professional growth, and efficacy. In addition, this chapter has focused on getting teachers to feel a performance investment in their work and profession. I have noted how important group skills are in making this happen, and have looked at how groups can be examined objectively. I have argued for the consultant to try to smooth relationships between teachers and principals as part of a general effort to ease teacher burdens.

5

Support Staff

Support staff are often neglected by professionals in the schools because they do not play as direct a role in education as do teachers, counselors, and administrators. Support staff include secretaries, custodians, nurses, lunchroom and classroom aides, security guards, and the like. Although they are often called "ancillary," their critical role makes them anything but that.

The consultant seeking entry into the school must understand the culture and be able to penetrate it if he/she hopes to create change. The support personnel are a key part of the culture, and their knowledge of the building, teachers, and students can be valuable. They can open doors for the consultant who wants to deal with teachers or administration, or they can be consultees themselves. They are important because they are on the front line.

Although some of the ways to help support staff may seem rather obvious, it has been my experience that special services personnel do not always put into practice many of these suggestions. Vinnicombe (1980) found, for example, that managers spend little time on secretarial development, a phenomenon that I have observed with other support personnel as well. Perhaps in our self-absorption with our own pressures, we often ignore or take support personnel for granted.

NEEDS OF SUPPORT STAFF

The consultant who helps support personnel meet their needs may be helping them to survive in their jobs, in a time of cutbacks and layoffs. According to Maslow's (1954) hierarchy of motivation (discussed in Chapter 3) the need for economic survival is at a fairly basic level (incorporating the *physiological* need for food and the *safety* need, for shelter).

Once their basic needs are assured, support staff often seek Maslow's third level: *belongingness and love.* They need to feel a part of what is going on in the school, be valued as important, and be included in team activities and decisions. Many support personnel feel disenfranchised and were themselves turned off by their own schooling experiences.

Support staff have strong *esteem* needs (Maslow's fourth level): to be recognized and valued for their specific skills and contributions as well as for themselves as individuals. The need for ownership of projects (discussed in Chapter 2) relates to this need for esteem. In the professional atmosphere of schools, aides and custodians are often viewed as low on the power and prestige scales. They have difficult jobs, some of them are paid poorly, and they receive little recognition. Even nurses and secretaries, despite their training, are sometimes out of the mainstream of the school process. They find that they have little to do with day-to-day decision making, and therefore it is harder for them to feel ownership of school projects.

The highest level of need in Maslow's system is *self-actualization*, the full use of one's abilities and interests. For support staff, we must look at how that can be achieved.

Another way to understand support personnel is to look at vocational personality themes (Holland, 1966). Holland identified six themes: realistic, investigative, artistic, social, enterprising, and conventional. Most applicable to support personnel are the realistic, social, and conventional themes. (Of course, not all support personnel fit such descriptions, but they can be useful.) *Realistic* people (often those working in the custodial, maintenance, and security roles) need to have concrete results for what they do. They enjoy work with tools and equipment and tend to be rugged, adventurous, and tough. *Social* types in the Holland scheme enjoy helping people. Aides and nurses are likely to be high on the social theme. Secretaries are typically characterized by the *conventional* theme, which values detail work. Such people want to be an important cog in the system rather than carry the responsibilities of leadership. They prefer to avoid conflict and theorizing. People of the conventional type want predictability in their lives in terms of hours, pay, and job duties. They do not like departing from established routines. In this regard, they also resemble the realistic personalities, but they are far less adventurous than the latter.

Another way of looking at support staff is to examine their coping styles. Vinnicombe (1980) developed a "typology of secretarial styles"

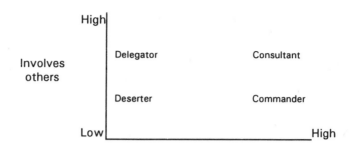

FIGURE 5.1. Typology of secretarial styles. From Vinnicombe (1980). Copyright 1980 by S. Vinnicombe and Avebury Publishing. Reprinted by permission.

similar to the managerial grid of Blake and Mouton (1964). The vertical dimension of Figure 5.1 illustrates how much secretaries involve others in their work. On the horizontal dimension, they are rated on their tendency to make decisions and take action. Perhaps other support personnel could be described in this way as well.

Vinnicombe describes the Deserter as a person who takes little action and does not involve others. The Commander, who possesses a more authoritarian style, is better at taking action but also does not choose to involve people in his/her work. Delegators are better at involving others but take little action on their own. The Consultant, perhaps ideal in many organizations, is capable of taking decisive action but chooses to involve others while doing so.

So we have come full circle. Many of the skills that make a good consultant also make a balanced support person. The consultant needs "consultant" support persons with whom to work. Consultants can work with their support personnel to develop decision-making, action-taking skills. If the consultant becomes more involved in their activities and helps them become more fulfilled on the job, it will make his/her work as a consultant easier.

PRESSURES ON SUPPORT STAFF

To cultivate support staff, the consultant must know the various pressures they face. Secretaries are asked to type letters for people from other departments, baby-sit disruptive students, be ambassadors to important visitors, type grant proposals with deadlines and standards for accuracy that are very demanding, and process attendance data promptly. They must find substitute teachers on short notice, struggle to learn computers and software, publish school newsletters and bulletins, and adapt to constantly changing department policies. Secretaries are expected to be able to respond to a multitude of demands, from clerical to social, to executive. For this, they receive a lower salary than their friends in business and industry and even less status.

Consultants can unwittingly add to the pressures a secretary faces. The consultant should help the secretary develop priorities. Many conscientious secretaries lose work time trying to do too much. A meeting with the secretary to determine the most and least important of his/her tasks, so that they can be done in an orderly manner and still satisfy his/her superiors, can be beneficial not only to the secretary but to the consultant as well, in that the consultant has made an ally in the office and has ascertained to what extent the secretary might be available for other responsibilities.

If a secretary is often out sick, it may be because he/she is struggling with an unreasonable workload. By observing the secretary's absence pattern, the consultant may be able to determine whether it is related to work stress.

Another means of diagnosing pressures that face secretaries and other support personnel is to analyze the signs and pictures they usually have on their desk. One such sign shows a person breaking up into hysterical laughter, with the caption: "You want it WHEN!? Such a staff member may be besieged by demands from many people, all of whom want their work done immediately. "TGIF" (Thank God it's Friday) signs may indicate that a secretary is so overworked or uninterested in his/her job that he/she cannot wait until the end of the week. Although such signs could indicate that the support person just has a sense of humor, the consultant should always be alert to the unconscious message.

A secretary could even be pressured by equipment that is poor or does not work. The consultant's ability to get through to administration to achieve a repair or to requisition some supplies may easily accomplish what some secretaries feel is an overwhelming task. Remember, if the secretary is characterized by the conventional personality he/she may dislike such assertions. However, Vinnicombe's consultant or commander type might relish such outreach.

Nurses' pressures include medical emergencies, suicidal cases, and student pregnancies. They have to report incidents of abuse and must tread the fine line between maintaining student confidence yet keeping parents informed.

Security people have to deal with the most difficult students, often risking their own physical safety. They have to enforce rules that may be inconsistent and are not always backed up by administration. These personnel often come under Holland's realistic personality. Wanting quick results, they are not always prepared for the negotiation and tuning in to student personality nuances, more characterized by the social theme.

Lunch aides are expected to discipline students and generally control them in what usually is an unstructured setting with unclear guidelines for student behavior.

Classroom aides are expected to know how to manage difficult students and help teachers with challenging remediation tasks, and they often find menial chores dumped upon them, such as changing diapers of profoundly challenged children, transporting piles of textbooks, or scoring repetitive worksheets.

Custodians cope with one emergency after another with limited budgets (and yet no one is ever satisfied with the physical state of a school building, especially in older, inner-city districts). Understaffing and budget problems prevent prompt response to all the requests. Equipment breaks down and there is pressure to fix it immediately; students have accidents that require quick cleanup.

USEFULNESS OF SUPPORT STAFF

The consultant who can tune in to the needs and pressures of support staff is in a unique position to enter a school culture. The roles and usefulness of support staff, as well as suggestions for entry, are considered here.

Secretaries

Vinnicombe's (1980) studies of secretaries indicated that they felt underutilized. (I have observed that this is true for all support personnel.) The consultant can help secretaries become successful, feel satisfied, and feel valued. Although such goals are appropriate for anyone with a secretary, they are very important for the consultant because the secretary is a key access route to entry. I have cited the critical roles of principals and supervisors in achieving entry. However, the road to the principal and supervisor leads through the secretary's desk. The gatekeeping role is a critical one for secretaries (Vinnicombe, 1980). They guard and protect the people for whom they work (if there is a good supervisor–secretary relationship). Figuratively, they have the "key to the castle." They can decide *who* gets to see the principal or administrator, *when*, and for *what reasons.* At some schools, secretaries *literally* have the keys: the authority to give consultants keys for rooms they need. Even with sanction for a consultation project coming from the superintendent, a poor relationship with secretaries will surely bog down the consultant's work. Secretaries have their fingers on the pulse of the school and usually know, more than most others, what is going on, who is doing what, and who are the people one has to know to get through to upper administration.

Secretaries' roles can be divided into *mechanistic* (typing, word processing, transcribing, recordkeeping) and *organic* (managerial, people-relating, problem-solving) tasks (Vinnicombe, 1980). Each function is critical to the consultant's success. How students and parents are received is important to the outcome of consultation and even to the effectiveness of the special education program. Are students and parents treated with respect? A consultation project involving parents is in trouble if the parents are not well treated when they come in or call. If parents become turned off by a frustrated or overwhelmed secretary, their lack of cooperation with teachers in the special education program can hurt the effectiveness of that program. Reports not typed on time can hold up conferences related to consultation and individual educational plan (IEP) purposes.

The following questions identify some of the consultant's needs that a secretary could be instrumental in meeting.

Are you notified promptly if someone comes to see you?
Can you get rush work typed? Will you receive telephone messages?
Can you find out what important projects are being worked on in the school office, so that you can develop consultation ideas?
Is it easy for you to obtain student records?
Can you quickly locate students or teachers with whom you need to work?
Will the secretary page people, or if that is not possible will he/she give you access to student and room schedules?
Will the secretary look up information on the computer database for you?
If the secretary talks to others in the school, does this factor positively influence your reputation as a special services team member or consultant?
Is your checking in and out of a building a pleasure?
Can you find out what key problems the school faces?

If the answer to any of these questions is no, the consultant should examine how effectively he/she has been cultivating the secretary.

Nurses

Nurses also face difficult tasks. They cope with epidemics and the medical neglect which often accompanies poverty and do physical exams for hundreds of students who participate in team sports and job programs (for working papers). Their knowledge of a family's socioeconomic level or stresses can be valuable to a consultant who is taking an ecological approach to a consultation. Nurses' awareness of medical and psychological issues relating to a student's athletic team participation may inform the consultant of the student's strengths and weaknesses. Their picture of teacher referral patterns to the health office may clue the consultant in to teachers who overindulge or are too strict with students about health issues. They know how well families cooperate in obtaining glasses or hearing evaluations for children. Nurses often have emergency telephone numbers to help the consultant contact a hard-to-reach parent. Nurses know the suicidal children, those who have recently returned from hospitals, psychiatric centers, or substance abuse treatment programs, and those who have been injured in fights. This is all critical information for the consultant attempting to help teachers manage students, and can provide valuable clues for areas of consultation entry (e.g., if statistics on students injured in fights are high). If consultation takes the form, say, of helping students cope with parental abuse, psychological pressures, or peer instigation to fight, the nurse is there to provide key support and information.

Caplan (1970) wrote extensively about his consulting with a visiting nurse's association. The similarities between problems faced by school nurses today and visiting nurses then are striking even though more than 20 years have passed. He noted that consultants may have to deal with the emotional pressures of nurses, including those who have made mistakes in their dealings with patients. He suggested working to improve nurse productivity in a culture that is in transition from authoritarian to participatory in terms of leadership (a trend we find now in the schools as site-based management takes hold). He also suggested increasing feedback from central policy makers to line nurses. He felt that consultants should try to facilitate the participation of nurses in policy making (when in schools they have little impact on policy). This can have an impact on the nurses' needs for belonging-ness and can increase their esteem.

Nurses can provide an opening for the consultant to deal with teachers or administrators, or they can be consultees themselves. Consultants interested in remediating reading problems could work with nurses to develop close vision screening. Such work may be more exciting and challenging for nurses than the routine physicals and complaints they usually deal with. The consultant should consider including the nurse as a group counseling partner in a Level I or II intervention. Groups could be formed to help pregnant students or to prepare teenage fathers to cope with births and childrearing.

One role of the consultant is to run interference for teachers in dealing with administrators. This task also applies to support personnel. By making administrators more aware of nurses' needs, for example, and by helping nurses gain the communication and political skills to obtain what they need from the principal and others, the consultant can enhance the effectiveness (self-actualization) of nurses and other personnel.

Lunch Aides

Lunch aides can be key allies and need to be appreciated by the consultant. They can provide critical family information about children, tell the consultant how students eat and play and what kind of peer interaction they have, and, with the consultant's help, construct a sociogram of a class's interaction patterns. They will tell you who the bullies and victims are and might have student management suggestions. One lunch aide identified a frequent gambling problem in a high school student who was rarely found in class but was in school every day. The reasons a student cuts class can be quite varied, so the insight gained from such information can pinpoint possible interventions. Another student cutting class told a lunch aide that he had to care for his baby in the afternoons, a common reason for absences in the inner city.

Lunch aides are often the first to see patterns of eating disorders, which are on the increase in teenagers. Although clinical intervention must take place with such students, at least another opening for systemic consultation has been made. The consultant can develop inservice programming on eating disorders (Level IV), train teachers to recognize the symptoms (Level III), and perhaps even have an impact on school curriculum (Level IV) to increase student awareness and build self-esteem around body image. In Chapter 2, I discuss a program to help lunch aides gain skill and increase their sense of belongingness and esteem.

Classroom Aides

Classroom aides also have valuable knowledge about students. They can help individualize work for students, implement behavior recording, fill out rating scales on student behavior, bring students to the consultant, talk to parents, and relate inside informtion about the student. They can relieve the teacher of burdensome tasks so that the teacher can follow through on recommendations from the consulting process. They can also help a teacher follow through on consultation interventions.

Aides need proper training to develop skills to change behavior. Schmuck (1982) tells of a program he developed to improve organizational functioning. Working at Meyers's Levels III, and IV, he taught aides, nurses, janitors, and even cooks, problem-solving and communication skills critical to effective organizational functioning.

They role-played the skills with each other (Meyers's Level III) and worked to change their own attitudes about communicating and problem solving. At Level IV, the consultant had an impact on program and across staff lines. With skills such as these, the support staff could become great assets, but such training takes time, commitment, and effort.

Security Guards and Attendance Officers

Security guards and attendance officers are often overlooked as resources. It is unfortunate how often consultants assume that guards are not educated or that they have nothing to offer, when in fact the opposite is more likely to be true. Many, regardless of formal education, have valuable insights into issues of student behavior and school change. Some guards I have known had themselves acted out when they were younger and could see through the manipulations of the antisocial student. At some schools, their responsibilities include transporting students, visiting homes, and otherwise providing logistical support, which can be utilized by the consultant who wants access to students and parents. Consultation projects could involve training security and attendance staff in effective communication with students (Meyers's Levels II and III) or in violence-reduction techniques (Level III). I have cultivated attendance and security staff relationships, and often they become a source of referrals of at-risk students. Security personnel are also invaluable for suicide prevention programs because they are in a position to see which students seem vulnerable, particularly to victimization by others.

Custodians

Custodians should also be cultivated. They can find the consultant a room to conduct consultations and can locate spare equipment or furniture. They too know many of the students. They can be assets in finding work for older students. Consultant's are always hard-pressed to find alternatives to classifying disruptive students under special education. Custodians and security people, who are mostly male, can provide masculine role models for boys who are without fathers. They can be an important resource, especially in elementary or junior high schools where there are fewer male teachers.

At one of our schools, the special services team utilized custodians to organize work activities to motivate students who needed hands-on experience. They provided physical activity for hyperactive students and created respect for the physical aspects of the school environment. Meyers's Level IV was involved because the activities required a program change and administrative approval. The actual contact between the custodians and the students was a Level II intervention. Intervention at Level III (which we did not do) could have helped the custodians be more effective in their communication with young people and educated them in basic principles of behavior change. Such a work program can sometimes ease custodian's pressures by providing an increased labor force. It may appeal to their belonging-ness and esteem needs if they become valued by the professional consultant and receive recognition for their efforts.

PROVIDING RECOGNITION AND STATUS

One guerrilla tactic (T. Jackson, 1977) for consultation entry is to provide some of the recognition and status support personnel need. The consultant should make eye contact and refer to support staff by *name*. I have seen some special services personnel and consultants walk into a school building and (without even a "please") order a secretary to find them a student or a custodian to get them a room. They expect compliance, perhaps because of their degree, position, or inflated view of themselves. Such people often end up talking to the wall. Support personnel can make the consultant's job a pleasure if the consultant gives them their due as human beings. If the consultant does not, he/she may find that many are skilled at stonewalling (passive–aggres-sive behavior). They may decide to be too busy to hear the consultant or may verbalize their assent and then not follow through.

It is also important to remember that support personnel have roles and lives other than in the school. Finding out about them can be an valuable step toward developing a good relationship. Furthermore, showing an interest in support staff's work, and praising it if appropriate, can be very rewarding. We all need praise, and although many of us know about the principles of reinforcing behavior that we want to see continued or increased, we often neglect to notice when someone has done a quality job. Appreciation, perhaps in the form of a written "thank you" when you hand material back to a staff member, or a comment on how difficult it must be to juggle all of his/her tasks, goes a long way toward creating alliances. Vinnicombe (1980) found that even satisfied secretaries felt they needed more "please" and "thank you" feedback. In sum, consultants should treat support personnel like they would want to be treated.

Taking on work from other departments was one point of dissatisfaction Vinnicombe, reported in his studies. Even if consultants have authority over a secretary, they may need to give him/her leeway in arranging tasks so that he/she feels more in control and has a sense of ownership of the job (Vinnicombe, 1980). Most support staff like to grow and expand. Special services personnel need to work at giving them status to meet their esteem needs. Vinnicombe (1980) also discussed the secretary's need to feel a personal identification and involvement in his/her manager's work. The consultant should share with secretaries something about the work he/she is doing and ask their advice about how to approach the consultation project. The secretary may then begin to develop "ownership" of the project. Besides creating status, this ownership also will translate into access to administration and increased cooperation in making a project happen.

Involve support personnel by asking for advice in dealing with the principal or supervisor. Such involvement may help a commander type of secretary and may motivate others who are less task-involved too. A secretary once informed me that a certain principal always wanted to be notified in advance of my coming into the school. This principal did not like "drop-ins."

Find out what support personnel see as the principal's and supervisor's priorities. They know the pressures principals face and may give the consultant clues as to why a principal is busy or feeling hasseled. One principal was too busy to see me one day. His secretary told me he was preparing a program for upcoming visits from student teachers. Because I had this information, I was able to offer to orient the student teachers to the role of the special services team in consulting to teachers. This saved the principal some time and was a valuable supplement to the training of these college students. It would not have happened without the cooperation of a secretary willing to share her supervisor's agenda for the day. It is also noteworthy that the principal never considered this a function of a special services team, so he never thought to ask us himself. This example illustrates how gatekeeping by a secretary can provide a positive opportunity for consultation entry.

Consultants can help support staff develop status by praising them to their supervisors in writing for the aspects of their jobs they do particularly well. One secretary was shocked and pleased at a letter I had written, as it was the only one of a positive nature that anyone had ever placed in her personnel file, despite that fact that she was viewed by most as a quite capable employee. I recently wrote a note to a custodian with a copy to the principal thanking him for his help in setting up a room for an inservice program. He had worked many years for the school system and told me this was the first time he had ever received a written note of thanks.

Mentioning a support staff member's help in the school newsletter also can be greatly appreciated. In bureaucratic environments, such niceties are often neglected. Recognition and increased status also can be facilitated by involving support staff in planning meetings for management of students, such as IEP conferences (see Chapter 2).

Teach new skills to increase status. Vinnicombe's studies indicate that secretaries often felt they were not applying their abilities to the fullest. I trained one secretary in a word processing program, who then increased her status by becoming the computer consultant for other secretaries. Secretaries can also gain status by learning to work with clients (e.g., administering paper-and-pencil tests to parents and students). They may enjoy becoming a part of the clinical team.

In summary, I have noted some key support staff who should be cultivated in order to make consultation more feasible. These include secretaries, nurses, custodians, aides, attendance staff, and security guards. I have reviewed some of their roles and needs and the pressures they face and discussed the access they offer to information about school functioning and students. I have noted how knowledgeable they can be, and have emphasized that recognition of their contributions should not be taken for granted or overlooked by the consultant.

If the consultant takes time to get to know the support staff (which often their own supervisors neglect to do), it will be appreciated and will pay off in consultation access. If the consultant shows a little sensitivity and gives support staff some investment of time, they can become important allies. The time spent cultivating support staff will be repaid abundantly, and consultants will find many openings to the inner school culture they never imagined were there.

6

The Parents

The consultant seeking entry must utilize every possible contact, including parents. Parents, as taxpayers, are your employers (Trachtman, 1981) and need to be treated as such. This means involving them in decision making, respecting them, and conveying to them a general feeling that they contribute to the school (Lambert, 1981; Remer, Niguette, Anderson, & Terrell, 1984). Christenson and Clearly (1990) cite Seely's view that student learning takes place only when there are productive relationships among all the participants in the educational process. They assert that education today is not progressing because of the separation of home, school, teachers, and students. They argue for an "effective parent–educator partnership to make school consulting effective" (p. 219).

MEYERS'S MODEL IN WORKING WITH PARENTS

In this chapter, I show how Meyers's model of consultation and the holistic approach can help facilitate parental involvement. I discuss how such involvement can be helpful to the school and consultant. Parents' needs, including to be informed about their children, to feel a connection with teaching and other school staff, to communicate with school administrators, and to have a role in their children's education, are looked at in the terms of the hierarchies of Maslow (1954) and others. Parents have often been denied the opportunity to participate in their children's educational programs (Simpson & Poplin, 1981; Weiss & Edwards, 1992; Huebner, 1992a). One task of the consultant is to change that through systemic and behavioral methods. Group approaches to involve parents are also explored here.

According to Meyers's consultation model, involvement with parents is primarily at Levels II and III (indirect service to the client, and service to the consultee–parent). At Level II, the consultant works with parents to modify the student's behavior by teaching the parents management techniques or by finding a way for parents to reinforce what the school is trying to accomplish.

A Level III intervention could include parent counseling around family tensions or frustrations or perhaps helping parents with financial and housing problems. It is also possible for a Level IV intervention to occur with parents if the parents have influence in the school or community. Examples include a Level III change in family structure if a father starts to take responsibility for tutoring his daughter; parental influence on PTA policy to support new school programs (Level IV); or parental participation on committees or in programs supportive of special education (Level IV). Meyers's approach helps the consultant *target* where to intervene with the parent. When the consultant is forced to think about Meyers's various levels, he/she can consider alternative interventions and be more focused when choosing them.

MEETING PARENTS' NEEDS THROUGH A SYSTEMS APPROACH

The problem of applying a structure such as Meyers's to the consultant's work with parents is that one could either view the family as its own system or as part of a larger system. The larger system could include the school and district and the immediate and extended community, as well as the child. Figure 6.1 illustrates the complexity of interactions possible. It is adapted from the "ecomap" of Knoff (1984) which was based in part on Bronfenbrenner's (1979) conception of the multiple levels of influence that act on a child (or on which the child acts) directly and indirectly. Knoff diagrammed Bronfenbrenner's description of four levels of systems that directly or indirectly involve the student: microsystem, mesosystem, exosystem, and macrosystem. These systems, in effect, form a kind of entry "map," a means of planning how to serve parents as well as other consultees. The consultant, wishing to improve relations with parents, may want to use this schema to target interventions. Although I use this to illustrate the variety of ways in which service to parents could be provided, such a typology could be applied to all aspects of consulting with schools and other organizations.

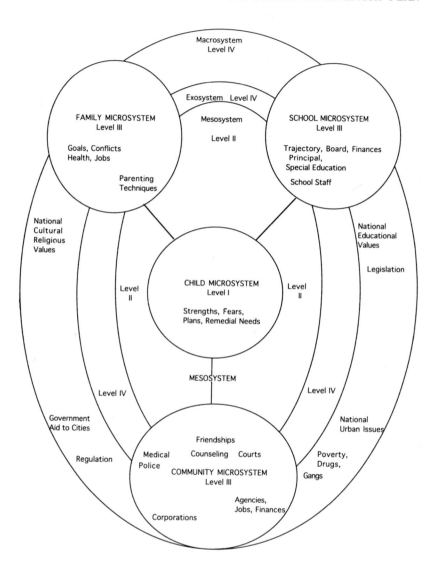

FIGURE 6.1. Systems impacting on the child: Consultation intervention targets. Adapted from Knoff (1984, p. 87), Copyright 1984 by Clinical Psychology Publishing Company Inc., Brandon, VT, and Howard Knoff. Reprinted by permission.

In Figure 6.1, each small circle is a microsystem within itself, although the one we are most concerned about is that of the child and its interactions with all the people and organizations that have an impact on it. The child brings to the system plans and fears, conflicts and interests, and so on. The family as a microsystem has its own conflicts and structure. Its working patterns, health, and goals will affect how it relates to the other systems. The school brings to the system its internal microsystem relationships and problems with staff, finances, board, and various departments. Finally, the community, from hospitals to police–neighborhood interactions, is represented within its microsystem.

Included in the child microsystem is the immediate sense of his/her experience: classroom, feelings about peers, roles played, values internalized from home, behavior in group settings, and so forth. The mesosystem involves any interaction in either direction between the microsystem of the child and the other microsystems: the child moving into a new school, being involved in community psychotherapy, or arguing with parents about doing homework. All these are mesosystem events. Another example might be a meeting of the special services team, the child, and a regular education teacher. The child interacting with peers at school is also a mesosystem event.

One important task the consultant has is to teach parents how to use the mesosystem. Parents need skills to maximize the attitudes and services of the various microsystems so they can serve the parent and child. One uses the mesosystem by learning to reach into other microsystems, making contacts, learning the language of those systems, and learning how to get around within them. The consultant who deals with parents must sensitize and educate them about how to be successful when dealing with each microsystem, whether it is their own child or other families, school, or community.

The exosystem consists of settings that do not directly involve the immediate microsystem, in this case the child, as an active participant, but in which events occur that affect the microsystem or on which the microsystem has an effect. A meeting between a consultant and a regular education teacher *about* a child occurs in the exosystem. Interactions between the microsystem of the family and the microsystems of the school or community are exosystem events. Exosystems also include the family and its relationships with the community. These could include a mother's connections with a local church, a father's relationship with an employer, or parents going for marital therapy to a local clinic or private therapist. When the child becomes *directly* involved in the therapy or medical treatment, or in a social agency's dealings with that child, the mesosystem is invoked. The consultant needs to look at the various exosystem happenings and help parents find a way to draw them into becoming mesosystem events, which then can directly benefit the child's microsystem. By doing so, one is using Meyers's conception of a Level IV intervention to make the system work better in general or for the child specifically. For example, a parent's involvement with a local church, synagogue, or mosque might be examined to see whether it could benefit or support the child.

Exosystem events may also include state or federal legislation, school board actions, and parental and school interactions with their own home and community contacts. These events also affect how family members, school, and community staff deal with the student. A mother's argument with an employer takes place in the exosystem, as does a father's negotiation with the Social Security Administration office or the courts. When a child's teacher is challenged by her own teenage son, it occurs in the exosystem relative to the identified child. Although none of these events directly affects the targeted child, the participants may carry with them the effects of these interactions when dealing with that child.

The macrosystem, which is overlapped by all the microsystems (except the child) because they influence each other, comprises the overarching societal influences: cultural attitudes, immigration patterns, the state of the economy, and political and world factors such as election-year priorities and promises, international conflict, recession, and each of these items' effect on schools and families. The macrosystem is reflective of cultural similarities, such as common problems and characteristics of urban schools or of Latino Catholics. Macrosystem events also affect consultation but are less accessible to the consultant for direct intervention. Rather, they offer a context for gaining a greater understanding of the influences that may affect the consultation. For example, new legislation to make it harder on aliens may indirectly affect how the consultant decides to interact with an immigrant parent and child.

This way of viewing the systems that have an impact on child, school, and consultant suggests clearly how ripe the opportunities are for expanding consultation with parents and other targets in a holistic manner. Figure 6.1 also indicates how complex and difficult it is to do so, because any attempt to interact with one part of the system has an impact on the other parts, and vice versa. Holistic consulting may start with the microsystem of the child but attempts to expand the impact and services through the mesosystem to the exosystem where the family microsystem exists. Using this approach, the consultant works with the family to learn how to gain from the greater whole (the exosystems), while empowering the family also to have impact on the other systems.

In my adaptation of Meyers's model, when the consultant interacts directly with the child he/she is in the mesosystem and is at Level I. Meyers's Level I interventions target the child's system to make changes in the child's adjustment and coping skills. These activities also take place between the child and the community, school, and family in the mesosystem.

Usually when other systems have a direct impact on the child, the focus of consultation is at Meyers's Level II, or indirect service to the child. When the consultant attempts change in the relationships between the parents and their child, the work is between the child circle and the family circle (Level II) but also includes the school's influence. Work with individuals within the family circle to improve, for example, their understanding, skill, confidence, or objectivity (Caplan, 1970; Parsons & Meyers, 1984) is at Level III.

The school circle encompasses all of the within-school issues and interactions that could affect the child, and that offer targets for the consultant, usually at Levels II, III, and IV. This circle overlaps the macrosystem because schools are influenced by national legislation and societal values. Exosystem factors for the consultant to intervene on could be the level of teacher training and expertise in handling curriculum or student behavior. If the consultant finds ways to improve school finances or attempts to change the trajectory of the school in a more positive direction, the consultant is using Level IV interventions at an exosystem level. Mesosystem issues within the school circle might suggest how the school brings parents and students together for planning and problem solving, how the principal relates to students when conducting an assembly, or how teachers approach the disciplining of students.

The community circle is another microsystem that exists primarily in the exosystem, but overlaps the macrosystem because of issues shared with other communities. One macrosystem event we in New Jersey have been facing is the tendency for the State Department of Education to take over school districts that have not been successful. Such looming possibilities influence consultation with parents as well as with other targeted groups. The consultant usually has a better chance of influencing the exosystem, because the macrosystem involves greater complexities, such as the state's political climate. However, it may not be stepping too far out of the consultant's role to empower parents through facilitating a voter registration drive or a dialogue on the issues facing community and nation.

Exosystem (Level IV) interventions with the community microsystem might involve offering school consulting services to improve decision making in community agency meetings, so that parents could be better served. However, the consultant must first look at the interactions *between* the four systems and try to influence them. The family relating to community and schools are exosystem interactions in which Level IV consultation can take place. Here the consultant brings together the courts and parents, corporations and schools, medical services for families, and so on. Teaching parents to operate effectively with the elements of the community helps to empower them.

Special services personnel can also work in the exosystem at various of Meyers's levels to bring school and community circles together to serve parents and students. A Level II intervention might be to train employers to move into the mesosystem and learn to handle special needs students more effectively. A Level III intervention could be to bring school and community together for training in handling parental abuse or in crisis intervention. Developing crisis *policies* would move the intervention to Level IV. The consultant could target school and community at Level IV in an exosystem move to arrange family therapy services from a community agency to be provided at the school. Each of the above interventions could involve parents as well. For example, when training employers to handle special needs students, the consultant could teach those same strategies to parents or have them help develop the training curriculum (Meyers's Levels III and IV). Parents could be involved in the planning and training regarding crisis intervention programs, perhaps even to help organize in the community so that resources are available to the school during a crisis (Poland, 1993). Parents might be enlisted to set forth the guidelines for the kinds of therapeutic services they want from an agency coming into the school. Encouraging parents to serve on boards or committees of community agencies is an exosystem activity that can empower them.

The consultant could intervene in an exosystem activity at Level III (the school–family axis) to help parents who, for example, may lack understanding of the temperamental behavior of their 10-year-old learning disabled child..* A school program for parents could show how children with learning disabilities often cannot process too many instructions simultaneously. Parents who lack child-handling skills

---

*Bear in mind that using Caplan's (1970) term "lack" can imply a one-up relationship between the consultant and parent. Parsons and Meyers (1984) decry such a view and argue for stimulation of a growth process which is empowering for teachers and, I would add, parents.

could be helped to develop child management strategies, such as observing or communicating positive and clear messages for what is expected of the child or creating a clear area of security in the family's policies and discipline methods (Smith & Smith, 1976).

We could extend Caplan's (1970) model to parents who do not have the confidence to be effective with their children. Consultants in this situation may simply need to be supportive and encouraging of the parents' attempts to cope. On the other hand, teaching mastery of child management techniques also builds confidence. The consultant, looking at Figure 6.1, might bring in the local Association for Learning Disabilities from the community circle to help a parent cope with a child who has a learning disability. The diagram suggests that this agency could be utilized for indirect service to the child circle (Level II) or service to the family (Level IV) or the school (Level III or IV), depending on the information or services this agency can provide. The figure illustrates the many ways in which a consultant can try to empower the family.

Other family issues could include the need to be more objective when dealing with a child. In parents, this can manifest itself by overidentification with a student's failures or successes. It can show as transference in which the parent sees the child as a sibling or parent with whom unresolved conflicts still exist. Passive parents who grew up with a dominating sibling may react to their child's attempts to make demands as if the child were that dominating sibling. The consultant can work with the parent to help make discriminations, for example, as to how the present situation differs from that of the past. Facilitating communication between child and parent to foster this would be a Level II mesosystem intervention, but it becomes Level III if only parents and their perceptions are being worked with.

A caution here: Consulting with parents and families is *not* family therapy (Dowling & Osborne, 1985). There is no doubt overlap, but the consultant's role in working with families is to help them function more effectively in support of the child and the school, and vice versa. Consultation avoids diagnostic labels and requires a more equal, collaborative relationship in which parents are involved in the problem identification, problem analysis, and intervention process, as well as later evaluating what was done (Valentine, 1992). Shared information and decision making are key aspects of a truly collaborative relationship between school consultants and parents (Christenson & Cleary, 1990). The school's responsibility to change its own microsystem as part of this dynamic process is another factor that differentiates this process from family therapy. Dowling and Osborne (1985) prefer that a relationship between parent and teacher be established *before* problems begin. This again makes family consulting different from therapy, as the consultant who facilitates this teacher–child–parent outreach is placed in a preventive role.

In a previous example, I cited an ineffective parental response (treating the child as if he/she were a dominating sibling) in dealing with a child's demanding behavior. The consultant could help this parent define clearly what is demanding behavior, record the frequency of the behavior, and explore alternatives to the ways in which the parent responds to the child's demands. This intervention can be expanded from behavioral to systemic by coordinating the teacher's and parent's approaches, which may help the parent see that there are other ways of interpreting or handling the demands, and extends the consultant's efforts into the school circle as well as the family circle.

Reframing can help the parent see that the child's behavior has meanings other than what is being *attributed* to the child; for example, a developmental stage in which the student needs to express feelings more openly in order to gain peer approval. A different parent's anger at the school could be interpreted as a sign of parental courage as well as love for his/her child. Students do not do as well in school when parents attribute their behavior to internal, stable, or global causes ("She's from a whole line of underachievers," or "He has an attention deficit disorder."). It is better to attribute behavior to factors that seem to be more modifiable ("She needs a different pace of instruction.") (Vanden Belt & Peterson, 1991).

Dowling and Osborne (1985) view children's problems holistically in the context of both school and home. They state that too often the school blames the child or family, and vice versa. They propose a problem-oriented, nonblaming "interactional" view that encourages the concerned parties to consider what each is up against. If a parent has to deal with a rigid principal, it is helpful to know what problems that principal faces within the school's microsystem (e.g., a group of teachers who undermine any innovative courses of action). This need to consider such additional and complicating factors is a feature of the holistic conception of consultation and cannot be ignored when trying to help parents solve problems.

Minor (1972) cites a case in which a student drew semipornographic drawings, which upset the teacher. A clinical approach (medical model) would have focused on the student's pathology. However, the consultant in this case took a holistic orientation and looked at the family *system*. The consultant discovered that the child was creating chaos to help the mother get rid of a boyfriend she could not openly reject. The boyfriend was increasingly upset by the problems the child was causing in school. The consultation involved work in the family microsystem with the mother on dealing with the conflicts she had over her boyfriend (Level III). This changed the ownership of the problem from the child to the mother. Mesosystem feedback from the teacher on the student's good and bad days helped the consultant know how to deal with the mother, so that the connection between the home conflict and the school behavior could be made. The triangle of the mother, her boyfriend, and the child being used to voice the mother's desires had to be understood before the child could be helped to reach her educational potential. Using the mesosystem triangle between the child, family, and school was the key to the solution. Minor felt that the environment in which a behavior takes place needs to be understood if the behavior in question (pornographic drawings) is to make sense. Such triangles need to be investigated if schools are to be more clinically effective with families (Johnston & Zemitzsch, 1988). They represent intervention at Meyers's Level III and also IV, because of the systemic involvement.

Consultation also diverges from the medical model because it views families in terms of their *strengths* rather than weaknesses (Shore & Vieland, 1989). Such strengths should be identified and listed in the family microsystem diagram (Figure 6.1) as important factors to use in consultation interventions. In this example, the child's mother might be encouraged to utilize strengths she has (Level III) in coping with her exosystem environment, rather than being dependent on her boyfriend to do certain tasks for her. She could be taught assertive problem-solving skills as a means of dealing more effectively with or getting rid of her boyfriend. She might be encouraged to utilize her vocational interests or specific job or hobby aptitudes to help her become more confident and independent. The consultant who builds on such strengths will be more successful in getting families to work on problems specific to them, as well as on general issues such as discipline or curriculum.

MEETING PARENTS' NEEDS THROUGH A BEHAVIORAL APPROACH

Some writers prefer a behavioral approach to involving families with schools. Behavioral approaches can be used in a holistic–systemic manner. Piersal (cited in Bergan, 1985) and Kratochwill and Bergan (1990) felt that consultants could help parents by teaching them to deal with student problems utilizing problem-solving behavioral consultation (PSBC) methods. When the methods are taught to both parents and teachers (Huebner, 1992a), who then work together to address the needs of the student, the approach is called conjoint behavioral consultation (Sheridan, Kratochwill, & Elliott, 1990; Sheridan, 1991; Sheridan, 1993). The idea is not only to act on the mesosystem by bridging the gap between home and school, but to maximize the treatment effect and promote generalization of the newly learned behaviors (by having the behaviors occur at home as well as in school). This exemplifies the holistic approach. Batsche (1991) has pressed for parents to be given supports such as those available to teachers in order to implement interventions.

In conjoint behavioral consultation, "problem identification" targets broader behaviors than in PSBC. This is because the behaviors are identified in the *context* of the situations that affect them *across* settings (home and school). The problem identification interview and subsequent interviews are conducted using semistructured interview forms and an active approach by the consultant. In problem analysis, basal data are gathered and analyzed and events at home viewed as antecedents for those at school, and vice versa. Sheridan called these cross-setting variables, which I believe affect the mesosystem. A treatment plan is created to intervene across settings, to enhance generalization, and to identify behavioral side effects. This is followed by evaluation (also done across settings).

Sheridan et al. (1990) wanted to see whether applying the conjoint approach was more effective in generalizing behaviors of increased socialization of withdrawn elementary students than consulting with the teacher alone. Targeting Meyers's Levels I and II, the consultants followed the conjoint behavioral consultation process. The data gathering and treatment implementation were in both school and home, which expanded the consultation to Meyers's Levels III and IV. Parents and teachers were interviewed and given comprehensive treatment manuals describing procedures, including goal setting by the student (this portion is shown in Figure 6.2). This goal setting increases student ownership of the problem, much as the cross-setting approach encourages parental ownership (Sheridan, Kratochwill, & Elliott, 1990).

Taped interviews were standardized and evaluated by observers to establish agreement on whether the goals of the interview were met. When a student set a goal, the parents and teachers would provide support and suggestions of behaviors that might be effective (e.g., establishing eye contact, giving a greeting, asking a question) (Level II). Students wrote up a self-report sheet and discussed the results with both teachers and parents (Levels I and II). Positive reinforcement was used.

Name: _____

Week of: _____

GOAL SHEET

With your teacher, decide on a goal that you would like to try to meet today. Your goal should be something that you can say or do with one or more new friends. Also, decide on a reward that you will earn by meeting your goal. When you think that you have met your goal, record it on your chart in the column "Did I Do It?" Complete the rest of the chart and show it to your teacher. After school, show the sheet to your parents, discuss your day at school, and set a goal for home.

	What was My Goal?	Did I Do It?	Who Did I Do It With?	When Did I Do It?	* * * * * * * *
M O N					
T U E					
W E D					
T H U					
F R I					

FIGURE 6.2. Goal sheet used in behavioral treatment programs. From Sheridan, Kratochwill, and Elliott (1990, p. 39). Copyright 1990 by the National Association of School Psychologists. Reprinted by permission.

A second phase helped students become more independent through self-monitoring, which was also reinforced (Levels I and II). Parents had their own checklist (Figure 6.3) to cue them as to which behaviors they needed to perform (Sheridan, Kratochwill, & Elliott, 1990). Parents and teacher communicated (Level IV, because the home and school microsystems were interacting through the mesosystem) via home–school goal sheets, written comments by both parties, and praise given at home and at school. Independent observations were carried

PARENT CHECKLIST

Name: _____

Date: _____

Directions:

At the end of each day, complete the following checklist. Specifically, indicate on the line to the left of each item whether or not you covered the content in adequate detail. If there are certain things that you are unsure of, please contact the consultant before continuing. The consultant will be available to provide feedback and suggestions. Thank you!

Goal-Setting

_____ Involved your child in setting a goal for neighborhood play situations.

_____ Your child could control this goal.

_____ Your child could be successful at this goal.

_____ The goal told your child what to do.

_____ The goal was very specific and concrete.

_____ The goal was recorded on the home chart.

Self-Reporting

_____ Inquired about play upon child's return.

_____ Inquired about goal attainment.

_____ Provided praise for positive, appropriate interactions.

_____ Allowed your child to record successful goal attainment on the goal sheet.

Positive Reinforcement

_____ Allowed your child to choose a reward to work towards when establishing the daily goal.

_____ Provided specific, genuine verbal praise for goal attainment.

_____ Provided the reward soon following goal attainment.

Home–School Communication

_____ Greeted your child and asked about his/her day.

_____ Reviewed your child's goal sheet.

_____ Praised your child for meeting his/her goal at school (if applicable), or encouraged your child to meet his/her goal the following day (if applicable).

_____ Prompted neighborhood carry-over (for example, encouraged your child to do similar things with a friend at home).

_____ Asked your child for neighborhood examples (for example, discussed alternative ways to initiate interactions at home).

FIGURE 6.3. Parent checklist for monitoring behavior. From Sheridan, Kratochwill, and Elliott (1990, p. 42). Copyright 1990 by the National Association of School Psychologists. Reprinted by permission.

on by consultants twice weekly (of both students in the study and matched controls), and a variety of rating scales were used to measure student progress from the start of the project to the end.

In the group in which the conjoint approach was used, social initiated behaviors increased both at school and at home. This did not happen at home for the students when consultation was with teacher only, despite school socialization improvement. Involving the parent helps to generalize results across settings and makes for stronger, more lasting treatment effects. However, Sheridan et al. note that such a conjoint approach takes more time and effort, and often parents are not easily involved because of logistics, because of the belief that such projects are the responsibility of the school, or because "we often [incorrectly] assume that parents have the skills to implement interventions without additional training" (Batsche, 1991, p. 2).

THREE KEY AREAS OF PARENTAL NEEDS

Support and Information

Parents need to have information. They want to be informed about their children, and not just when there is a problem. Viewed in the context of the needs pyramid (Maslow, 1954), once parental needs for basic physiological and safety requirements are taken care of, they are able to work for higher-level needs such as belongingness/love, esteem in the eyes of others, and, finally, self-actualization—the satisfaction that comes from self-development, learning, and personal growth. Consultants should particularly tune into the esteem needs related to the satisfaction that results from being recognized as good parents of achieving students. Unfortunately, in our society today, many parents are still caught up in basic survival, such as providing food (physiological) and shelter (safety) for themselves and their children. To be effective, the special services team member may have to help with those basic needs before parents can be partners in their children's educational program (thereby achieving such needs as belongingness and perhaps even self-actualization).

When I say parents, I refer to mother, father, foster parents, stepparents, and extended family parenting. Even in today's many single-parent families, I have found that fathers and extended family members are often available if asked. They are also rather pleased to be involved in school conferences, though they do not always expect to be. I once had a conference with the mother of a child in special education only to find out near the end of the conference that the father had also come but was waiting in the parking lot because he assumed the conference was only for the mother. I made it a point to go out and meet him and involved him in some of the decision making while he leaned out his car window. He was appreciative. Yet a study of father involvement in training parents to handle oppositional children found fathers involved in only 13 of 35 studies (Coplin & Houts, 1991). Building belongingness and esteem in fathers is a worthwhile goal of special services teams.

Consultants can also capitalize on the increased role of extended families in managing children. With proper releases, consultants can involve brothers and sisters, uncles and aunts, grandparents, godparents, and so on. Often these members of extended families have great influence over the child, and perhaps also in the community. Such influence can be channeled to help the child and school in ways the consultant alone could not. This is another application of the holistic concept, because the consultant must always be thinking about larger goals of school improvement when networking with family members.

Effective involvement of families takes time. This is another entry skill for consultation because building a parental constituency can open many doors in a school system. In the consultant's role as a counselor or monitor of special education students' progress, how much time does he/she spend with parents beyond mandated individual educational plan (IEP) meetings and the like? Borders and Drury (1992) urge greater parental participation in school counseling and education programs. Consultants should talk with parents about the good things that are happening: a high grade in a course or test, improved social relationships, or even an absence of disciplinary involvement. Consultants usually hear from the disciplinarian when a student they monitor misbehaves, but the consultant should also check with the discipline office and see whether a student is doing well, and if so report it to the parent. Zins and Ponti (1990) and Poland (1993) stress how important parent contact is when any problem comes up with a student. They suggest erring on the side of being conservative by involving a parent more than seems necessary.

If the consultant monitors children in special education, how often does the consultant sit down with a parent and discuss the strategies he/she and the teacher have developed to form the instructional guide portion of the IEP? The parent, knowing the student best, is in a good position to suggest means of coping educationally. Yet some researchers have noted that IEP meetings are characterized by inadequate participation by parents (Ysseldyke, Algozzine, & Allen, 1982; Ysseldyke, Algozzine, & Mitchell, 1982; Huebner & Gould, 1991). Some parents appreciate hearing about diagnostic data that indicate that their children learn only in small steps or need visual stimuli to make instruction more clear; knowing which reinforcers would work with their children; or learning whether their child responds better to firmness or to open-ended approaches. Here again, researchers have noted that parent conferences often allow insufficient time to discuss interventions (Ysseldyke, Algozzine, Rostollan, & Shinn, 1981; Huebner & Gould, 1991). Parents' needs for information often require greater time investment on the part of the special services teams whose goals include consulting (Huebner, 1992a).

Parents and teachers respond differently to consultants (Kratochwill & Van Someren, 1985). Parents even more than teachers may view the consultant as an authority figure. They may resist the consultant's attempts to work with them because they feel there could be an invasion of privacy, or even because of fear that family secrets may be discovered. In today's families, issues such as alcoholism; sexual, physical, and drug abuse; and even unemployment may be sources of embarrassment, and certainly not topics a family would automatically be open about with a special services staff member.

Silverstein (1991) found that parents were embarrassed by questioning done when case histories for special education classifications were being gathered, and that they saw little basis to feel pride in their handicapped children. (Such questioning often focuses on weaknesses rather than strengths.) Parents felt overwhelmed by the wealth of data presented in short time at IEP conferences, and upset by jargon and labels. The latter were often so disconcerting to parents that they were unable to absorb the meeting's substance.

Team meetings often engender strong negative emotional reactions in parents, yet many who feel this way do not express it (Silverstein, 1989). Such feelings can sabotage a consultation if the consultant is not aware of them. Most parents do not assert themselves at IEP meetings with educational specialists (Sarason, 1982), and often lack the knowledge to participate effectively in the IEP process (Skinner, 1991; Huebner, 1992a). To be effective, a parent must be able to explore curriculum options, teaching strategies, and behavior management techniques, among others.

Silverstein (1991) found that teams rarely provided parents with support, reading materials, or follow-up discussions. When they did, parents were most appreciative. They need to be involved as partners, not viewed as outsiders who have little to contribute. Skinner (1991) proposes that parents be oriented so that they can participate more knowledgeably, but also that the special services staff provide an "advocate" (p. 288), perhaps a school counselor or special education teacher who may be able to ask more cogent questions of the special services team and press them to use down-to-earth language as they present diagnostic data and program proposals.

Our special services team developed a parent feedback/satisfaction questionnaire (Figure 6.4) to determine whether parents really understood what went on at the IEP conferences and to give them an opportunity to express feelings about the conference using another medium. We hoped this would help parents feel that their reactions were valued. We often found that they really did not understand some of what was communicated, especially the meanings of classifications and of test results.

Connection with Teachers

Another important parental need, which relates to Maslow's belongingness and esteem needs, is to communicate with teachers. This is because parents need to feel a connection with the school and their children and also the potential esteem from being valued by the school for what they can contribute. Although the preceding behavioral intervention example (pp. 148–151) certainly can facilitate such communication, it is often not so easy for parents and teachers to get through to each other. When students are difficult to handle, there is often strain between parent and teacher. Teachers may feel insulted if the student implies a lack of respect for them, and they may quickly put parents on the defensive for not raising their children right. Typically, the universities do not train teachers in how to talk to parents (Sarason, 1982). Teachers often have perceptions of parents as deficient, or as having no other responsibilities besides the child (Christenson & Cleary, 1990). Christenson and Cleary state that the practices of the school seem to determine (more than parent characteristics) how much involvement there will be from parents.

Parents often wait for the school to involve them. To remedy this, the consultant must model, train, and/or play mediator. If parents view their participation as "directly linked" to their children's achievement, they are much more likely to participate actively in home–school efforts (Rich, 1987). This "bringing together" is a holistic mesosystem concept to expand the scope of consultation. One way the consultant can model effective conferencing behavior is to give teachers tips about how to talk with parents more effectively. For example, starting off parent conferences with at least one positive item about the student begins to break down parent–teacher misperceptions (Henderson, 1990).

PARENTAL SURVEY OF CHILD STUDY TEAM SERVICES

Parent's Name _____   Relevant facts _____

School _____   _____

Child's age _____

Instructions:

All the following questions are to be asked in an interview with a parent. Answers should not be Yes or No. Parent needs to give feeling–reaction input. This should occur at end of the IEP conference. If the parent doesn't want to answer, put in "no answer."

1. Did you know why your child was referred to the child study team?
2. Did the school explain the referral procedure to you during the Prereferral Parent Conference?
3. Did you receive and understand the letter about the referral?
4. Did you know you had a right to refuse permission for this evaluation?
5. Did you understand the results of the team's evaluations?
6. Did you understand your child's classification?
7. Whom would you contact if you had a problem with your child in the future program?
8. What suggestions do you have to improve child study services for your child?
9. What do you see yourself doing to help your child, educationally?

Answers: (Put down exact words and note any affects)

1. _____
_____

2. _____
_____

3. _____
_____

4. _____
_____

5. _____
_____

6. _____
_____

7. _____
_____

8. _____
_____

9. _____
_____

FIGURE 6.4. Parent feedback/satisfaction questionnaire. Permission to reproduce this form is granted to purchasers of *Entry Strategies for School Consultation* for professional use only.

In a related situation, at a difficult conference in which the family was called because of a student suicide threat, I saw anger, fear, and resentment on the faces of the three family members who came. They were tired of the school calling them about this student and felt ashamed and threatened. I started off the conference by emphasizing that although we were worried about their daughter, she was a fine student who was very well liked by the staff. There was relief and surprise on the faces of the family. They had expected to be blamed for the student's problems. I took pains to find out how they saw the situation, and when they pressed me as to why the student was suicidal, I made it clear that the causes were complex, and attempted to relieve them of blame. I focused on their needs and concerns, and eventually they began to share some of their family pain.

The consultant can help a teacher hear what a parent needs, and help the parent digest the teacher's concerns as well. The modeling of clinical skills (Huebner, 1992a) (a Level III intervention) can aid the teacher in being more effective in reaching parents. Face-to-face meetings with parents, teacher, and a special services staff member can often resolve disputes that started with teacher notes or calls to parents.

Parents, conversely, can help teachers with student behavior and achievement by working with students at home on tasks for self-improvement. Such tasks can include limiting television time, completing homework (Olympia, Jenson, Clark, & Sheridan, 1992) and increasing reading and conversational time (Walberg, 1984). Erion (1992) writes that few parents receive such tasks from the schools, yet cites a number of studies showing that parents can improve word identification through curriculum-based measurement probes, use of flash cards, and oral story reading by their children. Some parents will even come in to school to help with behavior modification projects that teachers do not have time to implement. However, when parents arrive at schools, they often become turned off because school personnel act as if *they*, not the parent, own the school (Sarason, 1982). Sarason stated that Public Law 94-142 mandated involvement of parents in special education programming, but a law alone could not create the *spirit* of real involvement. Rather than conceptualizing schools as identifying and treating problems in students, the consultant needs to take a developmental–system orientation that affirms the roles of home and community as well as school to help children develop (Christenson & Cleary, 1990).

Two parents with whom our special services team worked became annoyed with the school because their severely handicapped daughter failed to make progress in special education. They obtained a lawyer and launched a due process appeal. When the school psychologist involved them in conferences with school staff (i.e., facilitated access across the mesosystem), the dispute narrowed to differing interpretations of technical language, which were quickly ironed out. One of the disputes was around a physical therapist's microgoals of stimulating certain muscle groupings. The parents did not understand that such goals were important in the physical therapist's own microsystem and did not feel such methods were relevant to goals they had for mobility to accomplish specific practical tasks. The physical therapist agreed, after the consultant reframed the issue, to focus more broadly on the therapy, with the parents' goals as the priority. The consultant helped the therapist move out of his microsystem across the mesosystem and into the parents' microsystem to see why they had certain beliefs. The consultant also worked with the school so that interruptions to the therapies caused by the school schedule would be eased.

The parents did their part to implement the program revisions agreed on, which included increased stimulation of their child. The "enemy" was turned into an ally because the parents were empowered to have input, which previously had been frustrated. Because of the parents' influence in the community, there was a networking effect from this intervention. The parents were able to help the school obtain equipment (a Level IV impact on school programming) to further aid this student. As in Chapter 4, where the consultant spends time with teachers who are unhappy and critical, an investment of time with such parents will help cement a positive relationship between parents and school.

Henderson (1990) noted that schools need to reach out more. She suggested that schools provide child care when there are meetings, that parents be involved in policy development, and that meetings be more fun and less businesslike. She noted that the last thing busy, tired parents want is a "Robert's Rules of Order meeting" (p. 24). More of a partnership in agenda construction can also help, but it requires improving the *interaction,* not just increasing the amount of contact (Christenson & Cleary, 1990) between school and parents.

Communication with Administrators

Parents also have a need to communicate with administrators. These include principals especially, but also vice principals, central office administrators, and board members. Communication of this sort often falls under Maslow's (1954) belongingness need and is somewhat related to safety or survival needs, in that parents are protecting their children when they advocate for them with principals. Parents also have esteem needs when reaching out to administrators, as association with those in power is in itself a kind of recognition. Here again, special services personnel—already benefiting from a good rapport with the principal and other administrators, it is hoped—can become facilitators of positive communication. At an elementary school in our district, some parents were angry at a principal whom they felt was unresponsive. The school psychologist and learning consultant had coincidentally formed a group of parents to stimulate students' verbal skills and to help with general parenting issues. The parents who came to the group were some of those who were critical of the principal, and they were quite vocal. The group leaders reframed the parents' anger and criticism into specifiable goals, drafted a list of these concerns, and, with group permission, discussed it with the principal. She responded with specific steps to address the parents' concerns. The parents felt they had been listened to, and became school allies instead of critics.

The above is an empowering strategy. The hostility toward administrators was channeled, and the strong interest in the school and children, which motivated the hostility, was *reframed* into a positive activity.

Discipline policies in the school do not always reflect parental input, despite the fact that parents' needs to protect their children result in their deep concern about discipline issues. Effective discipline programs involve parents from the start in planning, developing guidelines and consequences, and helping the school implement the policy. This means that parents must be on school discipline committees both as individuals and as representatives of the Home and School Association (PTA, etc.). Parents can help schools find alternatives to the usual disciplinary consequences of detentions, suspensions, and the like. Schools can help parents see that changes in children's behavior can be made without the use of corporal punishment or loss of temper (Valentine, 1992). If there is a discipline committee in the school or district, the consultant should get involved and convince the committee to involve parents as well. Such involvement is a means of entry for the consultant and can help open the school to a greater sharing of purpose with parents. Henderson (1990) suggests that parents serve on other committees as well, and give input on curriculum changes, such as a new reading program.

PARENT SUPPORT GROUPS

Special services personnel have run parent groups for many years (Meyers's Level II and III) to improve management skills of parents or to educate them (Platt & Bardon, 1967). Groups help because they encourage parents to do concrete things to cope with their children. Thus, parents, with group support, are willing to do such tasks as count behaviors (Flanagan & King, 1980). There is some question as to whether workshops, readings, or learning prepackaged training programs such as Systematic Training for Effective Parenting (STEP), Parent Effectiveness Training (PET), and Active Parenting really produce change in parental behavior (Kramer, 1990). However, parents *like* such groups and their participation can be effective in advancing school achievement and behavior (Kramer, 1990).

Consultants need to take advantage of timing when planning group interventions with parents. For example, kindergarten parents are often the most readily available because many bring their children to school and pick them up. Aden (1991) talked with a group of such parents, all of whom wanted to be meaningfully involved with their child's beginning school experiences. She set up a group of weekly workshops called Parents and Teachers Helping Children to Succeed (PATHS). The group's goals were gleaned from talks with parents about their needs and by consulting the schools' mental health team, neighborhood centers, parent groups, and community resources. This meso- and exosystem approach (Level IV) holistically broadened the conceptual base of the group to include parent and community priorities. Topics ranged from helping parents understand the physical and psychological development of their children to helping them become knowledgeable about the computer terminology used in their children's education. Many of these were Level III interventions, as they dealt with parents' knowledge and skills. Refreshments were served, reminder notices sent, and speakers coached on how to speak to parents.

Aside from increased confidence shown by these parents, who largely came from public housing projects, the discipline problems in the kindergarten became almost nonexistent and student attendance improved. Aden also noted decreased misunderstandings between school and parents. My guess is that as parents' needs for belongingness and esteem were met by these groups, there was less anger and alienation. As parents' skills grew, some self-actualization needs no doubt were also met.

An idea for consultants who are concerned with prevention issues is to form parents' groups for divorcing adults to help them ease their children into the transition from intact to single-parent families (Bloom et al., cited in Gutkin & Reynolds, 1990) or to help parents aid their children in coping with loss.

Smith and Smith (1976) posit many good ideas for helping parents manage their children using a behavioral approach. This approach emphasizes building a sense of consistency, security, and predictability in children's lives—a strategy well-suited for the turbulent 1990s. They encourage child responsibility by having the student restate the prespecified consequence for misbehavior, as well as a consistent problem-solving, not blaming, approach, and they strongly support the parents' authority role.

PARENTS AS A CONSTITUENCY

The consultant concerned with entry strategies also sees the parent group politically: as a constituency (Sarason, 1988), as a resource in a time of increasingly limited resources (Sarason, 1982), as potential allies in the management of children, as a networking source to the community and its resources, and as voters for school budgets (which are under attack nationally as this book is being written). People do not mind voting for increased expenditures if they feel they are getting something for their money. It is my personal experience that citizens may be hostile to the schools because of their own negative experiences as students (see also Liddle, cited in Magary, 1967). Many voters feel disenfranchised, and therefore vote down bond issues and school taxes to express their frustration, which goes deeper than just the financial burden. They want to feel more a part of government in general and of schools specifically. They want to feel that government and schools can be more responsive. This lack of confidence in government and schools led to one of the biggest victories for Republicans in the New Jersey elections of 1991 (after a Democratic governor and legislature passed sweeping tax increases to better fund the schools).

Special services personnel can turn parents from critics to allies if they effectively utilize their relationship with parents through the student monitoring role. One formerly alienated parent who came in to learn child management techniques from the school psychologist became active in the parent–teachers association because she felt she would now be heard. It is easy to make allies of people if they feel someone values their feelings.

A more systemic (Level IV) example was cited by Snapp, Hickman, and Conoley (1990). A district faced a crisis of anger in the Mexican-American community because of concerns that their children were not being properly educated. Their school psychologist worked with the administration and board to improve communication with this key parent group. They held evening meetings with board committees on different topics such as achievement test scores, bilingual education, and the tendency to classify Mexican-Americans under special education disproportionately to their numbers. The ongoing dialogue cut through the hostitility and paved the way for improvements to be made.

Zigler, Kagan, and Muenchow (1982) cite Adams's finding that parents who help develop policy actually may themselves end up changing in a positive direction. This study also illustrates the importance of involving minority parents without being condescending to them (in order to "socialize them").

The consultant's attitude can make a difference too. The consultant is only one individual, but when parents call the school the consultant represents the entire school district to them. Sometimes the consultant might answer a parent's call but find that the parent wanted a different department. Perhaps the consultant is from outside and does not know where the parent should be referred. However, it is advisable to help the parent find the person he/she is looking for. Let parents know that consultants and special services personnel are there to be of help and the word may spread. In such a situation, consultants are doing public relations to promote their work but also reducing alienation by making sure parents receive personalized service, no matter how large the school bureaucracy may be.

ORGANIZED PARENT GROUPS

Organized parent groups are another source of alliance. Too often, they function without much school support, especially from professional special services staff. If consultants invest the time to go to these meetings and show interest, they may help parents feel more connected with the school. Consultants might offer to speak to these groups on an area of their expertise. That too can create openings to further involve parents in supporting consultation in particular and the school in general.

While working at a special school, I organized a career conference for students with learning disabilities and their parents. The conference brought in experts to help parents and students learn about how learning disabled (LD) students can cope with the career planning process, what services colleges provide for the LD student, and how employers deal with the LD student. The Level I intervention involved providing information and counseling to students; Level II assisted parents with methods for student planning, such as helping students to fill out applications or find financial aid; Level III involved teaching parents about learning disabilities and how colleges and employers deal with it; and Level IV brought in the community resources. This conference provided an excellent entry point for the consultants because the parents were highly motivated, being naturally concerned about their children's futures (safety and esteem needs). Parents volunteered to be speakers or to obtain them through their community contacts. Speakers were oriented to the needs of LD students (a Level III intervention) and trained to talk to them (Level II). The parents' *participation* consolidated the ally role, which later made them much more available to the special services team. Many parents consented to have their names listed in a career resource file and to talk to students about the work they do. Using parents to make actual programming changes in a school is a Level IV intervention. It also gives the parents a greater feeling of ownership of the school programs and of their children's education. The conference opened up the mesosystem, teaching students how to use the system to enter other microsystems or constituencies.

Newman (1967) tells how Dr. H. N. Blackwell, of the London, Ontario, schools tried to bring school and community together by organizing a workshop on teens for principals, guidance personnel, and mental health agencies. Our special services team did a similar project in a junior high school, but the workshop was for the teens themselves. We brought in experts on various teen concerns such as suicide, alcoholism, drug abuse, pregnancy, and so on, and held a 1/2-day workshop. We did not bring in parents and thus neglected an important opportunity to build a constituency.

One task of holistic consultation is to research parents' needs and find ways to meet those needs through the resources of the school or the special services team. Conversely, the needs of the school can be researched and parents considered for how they can help. When parents are enlisted to help, they, in turn, are helped because they become empowered. Needs can be uncovered through parent conferences, group meetings, parent–teacher associations, or questionnaires. Consultants find it hard to involve people if they are not aware of their needs. The consultant must determine these needs prior to moving ahead impulsively and pushing his/her own agenda.

In a similar vein, Scheinfeld (1979) utilized organizational development methods to improve classroom instruction. In doing so, the organizational development was *integrated with parental involvement* to bring an extra dimension into the picture. Parents, not just school or district staff, were considered targets of the approach, and thus were involved directly in group meetings about school change (see also Weiss & Edwards, 1992). In developing the organization, we must recognize that parents are truly a part of the school organization and can benefit from training and participation. The issue in both of the above examples is *inclusion*. Weiss and Edwards (1992) examined school signs and letters to parents to see if they promoted inclusion. When they saw they did not, Weiss and Edwards revised them. The use of organizational development within a school is a Level IV intervention, and so is bringing parents in to participate. Here the mesosystem is invoked, as the consultant works between the school and family systems.

SUMMARY

In summary, I have reviewed the use of Knoff's, Bronfenbrenner's, and Meyers's models as applied to systems and behavioral approaches to meeting parent needs and involving them more effectively in the schools. Such approaches can help parents feel more closely connected to teachers, communicate with administrators, and have a greater role in their children's education. When parents' needs are considered, and when parents, even those who are difficult, are included, students can be managed more easily, teachers do better and are recognized for their efforts by parents (Christenson & Cleary, 1990), and academic and behavioral problems show improvement. Support is then developed for the schools in general and for the consultant's projects in particular. Approaching parents through groups and the development of a parental constituency can accomplish much for the consultant, including the power to convince supervisors and principals to permit further entry for consultation. A community network is accessed, and a cooperative alliance between teachers, administrators, and consultant is built to help with individual issues of student management, as well as with more global issues of how to run a school more effectively.

III

BARRIERS TO ENTRY

7

Encountering Resistance

In a sense, this entire book is about resistance, because entry strategies serve to overcome barriers to consultation. However, this chapter attempts to pull together some of the key issues and solutions related to resistance. Issues to be explored here include (1) why and how resistance occurs at the organizational and individual level; (2) external factors that foster resistance; (3) how resistance manifests itself in the consultee; (4) voluntarism is an issue of resistance; (5) consultant issues that foster resistance; and (6) how to overcome resistance.

WHY RESISTANCE OCCURS

Resistance at the Organizational Level

Parsons and Meyers (1984) claimed that resistance often occurs because of inadequate contract negotiation or because entry has not been fully established. This may happen because the school did not clarify the problem clearly enough for the consultant or, the consultant did not assess the problem adequately (Zins, 1981; Zins & Ponti, 1990). Assessment depends on the problem's being clearly identified prior to intervention.

Resistance also often occurs because there is pressure to focus on interventions before proper data are gathered. The consultant may have thought that entry was established but really did not know the system, its readiness for change (Zins & Ponti, 1990), or how various system characteristics, such as the hierarchy, communications patterns, alliances, and the like, make it impractical to implement what appear to be good ideas on the surface (Sarason, 1982).

Sometimes the organizational setting has to be altered to make the consultee comfortable with consultation. Setting factors described by Bergan (1985) include the principal's behavior (see Chapter 2) and school system expectations (for class behavior standards, curriculum progress) (see Chapter 4). Another setting factor would be the degree of consultee involvement in the system in developing the plans for change (Zins & Ponti, 1990). Zins and Ponti said that all organizational members need to be involved in such decision making.

Consultation may also be casually or prematurely implemented (Huefner, 1988), which can cause resistance. Consultation intervention assistance programs often lack good descriptions of the specific procedures necessary to implement and carry them out (Zins, 1981; Zins & Ponti, 1990). Huefner (1988), writing about consulting teachers, stressed that such factors as unrealistic case loads, undertraining or overloading of the resource teacher (who may be new in the job), pressure to get the consulting teacher to tutor students instead of improving the regular education program in general, expecting consulting to be a panacea, getting inadequate support from regular educators, inadequate funding, and faulty assumptions about cost savings or program effectiveness all contribute to the potential for resistance to a consulting program. Neglecting any of these factors can inhibit entry. Huefner challenged the effectiveness and supposed cost savings for pull-in programs, indicating that more research and honest communication about the pros and cons of consulting are needed if consultation is to be sold to schools.

Consultants often do not plan how they will do program evaluation, nor do they always follow up adequately (Zins & Ponti, 1990). Since these issues can cause resistance, they must be resolved before intervening.

In order to establish entry, both outside and inside consultants need to know what kind of system they are entering. The outside consultant may more easily recognize the need to assess the organization than do inside consultants, who may take their system for granted and thus may not do careful diagnosis. Conoley and Conoley (1982) viewed entry into the organization as crossing a boundary. On the other side of the boundary are all the staff groupings and forces in the consultee system with which one has to contend. These become even more complex after entry is achieved, with multiple problem formulations, staff relationships, and the trajectory of the school as key factors.

All these factors help determine whether a system is proactive or reactive (Parsons & Meyers, 1984). *Proactive* systems are flexible and able to anticipate conditions that will occur and demands that are made on them. A proactive system is ahead on national developments, such as the regular education initiative (Hallahan et al., 1988) or the inclusion movement (to involve challenged children in regular classrooms regardless of severity of needs), and prepares to cope with such issues before they are forced to by external pressures, legislation, or regulation. *Reactive* systems are often already in crisis when the consultant is asked to intervene, because they are faced with state mandates or labor problems. This may make it somewhat easier for a consultant to enter but places great pressure on the consultant because of the need for quick solutions. The consultant entering a reactive system must negotiate a very clear contract as to realistic expectations and time frames. Zins and Ponti (1990) note that sufficient time is not always allowed for change to occur. Proactive systems are easier to work with but may be harder to enter because they see little need for the consultant. The consultant needs to sell his/her role as a facilitator and indicate how additional staff growth can be fostered. Perhaps the consultant could help improve school communication and efficiency even further. In a proactive system, assessment of school needs is even more important because those needs may not be very apparent to administrators of a well-functioning system.

Resistance to consultation manifests itself at the organizational level, according to Parsons and Meyers (1984), in the following ways:

1. *Desiring system maintenance.* The consultation process is seen as draining energy from a limited supply in the system. The system is being asked to make adaptations and expend energy. Here the consultant must find ways to reduce demands on the system. This could occur by using as much of the existing structure and procedures as possible: staff, forms, systems. The school must be shaped slowly without threatening the roles of key administrators.

2. *Seeing the consultant as an outsider.* This can occur even with an inside consultant if that consultant is operating out of his/her usual perceived role. For example, school psychologists are not seen as having much to do with outcome-based education because they are rarely involved in the planning sessions (Cobb, 1992). I have been interested in mentoring new teachers but have never been asked to participate in such planning because it is not seen as my role in the school. Consultants should become involved in school committees and projects if they hope to change that perception. I had to keep after the union representative in our school to be considered for a role in the mentoring program. In addition, consultants should dress more like the school staff, be aware of their history and philosophy, participate in as many school functions as possible even if they seem irrelevant (Chapter 4; see also Parsons & Meyers, 1984), and associate with the people on the staff who have status.

3. *Rejecting the new as nonnormative.* This is an extension of Sarason's (1982) concept of school regularities, in which any threat to the usual way of doing things is seen as alien. Consultation may be seen as conflicting with existing administrative structures and educational values (Dyck & Dettmer, 1989). The very bureaucracy that is typical of school systems presents a block to the effective collaboration and problem solving that can lead to educational excellence (Skrtic, 1991). If resistance to change is to be overcome, the consultant must respect time-honored practices, obtain both formal and informal sanctions, and try to make smaller changes. Small successes will encourage acceptance of the consultant without creating large threats (Kirpius, 1985).

4. *Protecting turf.* Changes in a reading program may threaten a Title I administrator. (See Chapters 2 and 4 for turf issues.) It is important to protect the security of people and their roles. In their book, Parsons and Meyers (1984) present a good exercise to practice identifying sources of organizational resistance (pp. 106–111). They suggest first writing a description of a recent consultation contract that did not work out well; second, guessing at the reason for the resistance; and third, trying to determine which of the above four forms of resistance this took. A fourth step is to look at the individual and organizational behaviors that might have provided a warning cue to this resistance. Finally one should review the entry process and try to figure out which changes in the initial interview, contract discussions, or actual contacts with various people might have reduced the resistance.

Some organizational behaviors mask resistance, whereas others, which look like resistance, may not be at all. A school district may appear to welcome the outside consultant because having a consulting program seems to be the appropriate thing to do. However, the district may not have thought out how it really wanted to use a consultant or properly oriented principals and other administrators. One such school district seemed easily open to a consultant, whereas a panel of administrators and staff at a second one grilled him mercilessly about his intentions (Meyers et al., 1979). In reality, the second district was the one most easily entered. The first district had not been prepared for consultation, but the second district, because of the well-thought-out questioning, was ready. As noted in Chapter 4, staff who appear hostile or challenging to the consultant may become the consultant's best allies because of their perceptiveness, investment in the process, and caring about the system and what happens to it.

When gathering data at the level of the system, one way to reduce resistance is to start with a less structured approach and later move to a more structured one (Parsons & Meyers, 1984). It is less threatening to do an unstructured observation just by walking the halls and trying to observe empathically and objectively. Parsons and Meyers suggest then increasing the structure through survey techniques based on hypotheses from the observations and interviews with administration to review survey results and to learn more about the elements, structures, and processes of the system; the forces acting on it; and the system's trajectory (where it has been and where it is going). Finally the most structured data gathering is focused observation, using objective scales to measure such factors as who talks to whom in the organization or how often various forms of communication take place.

Resistance at the Individual Level

Resistance at the individual level can be explained in part by looking at the individual's psychic "cost" versus any payoff that the consultee obtains from participating in consultation (Parsons & Meyers, 1984). The consultee motivated by (experiencing the cost of) aggravation from a student's behavior will look for various payoffs in consultation. These payoffs include receiving problem-solving service and gaining camaraderie. The former gives the consultant "expert power" (value that is attributed to the consultant), and the latter places referent value on him/her. Outside consultants often have the expert power but need to develop referent power, whereas inside consultants, who have had the chance to relate well to staff, may possess referent value but have to work to be perceived as experts, that is, to be respected for their knowledge and skills. The expertise of the consultant or teacher is likely to increase the strength of treatment or consultation (Gresham, 1991), as is the consultant's status (referent) level (Kratochwill & Van Someren, 1985). Hence, developing both expert and referent status is one way of overcoming resistance.

Parsons and Meyers (1984) say that consultees balance these payoffs against costs, such as: the time and energy they have to put into consultation; a fear of the unknown, which includes a potential for embarrassment; a fear of being criticized (there is sometimes a stigma attached to needing consultation); and a concern that maybe the costs may outweigh any returns.

Piersal (cited in Bergan, 1985) lists consultees' perceived costs, actual time limitations, and other demands on the consultant as elements that make regular, effective consulting difficult (see also Dyck & Dettmer, 1989). Consulting must be done regularly (at least once a week) to gain the confidence of staff (Newman, 1967). The consultant must be available to follow up on consultation or the consultee's confidence in that process will be lost. There is a kind of teacher wisdom that says, "This too shall pass," referring to the countless new programs that come into vogue and disappear without follow-up or continued support by the school administration. This applies to consultation, for teachers do not want to open up and be vulnerable to examination and change and then be abandoned. As Sarason (1982) noted, teachers will evaluate the changes a consultant wants to make based on their knowledge of the success of previous proposals for change in that school. Regularity of contact with staff and frequent follow-up are the remedies for such cynicism.

School crises, such as student violence, are also costs to staff. Consultee resistance breaks down when the consultant can contribute some *direct service* to the school (Newman, 1967) to lower those costs. For example, the consultant who can intervene quickly to help a school through a crisis often overcomes much of the initial resistance to entry (Meyers et al., 1979).

Another cost issue raised by Piersal (cited in Bergan, 1985) is that the consultee may feel pressure to move on with the curriculum or serve students other than the identified client who have been neglected. Consultation may be seen as an obstacle to this, with insufficient payoff to justify the effort (which is perhaps aimed at just one student). Although I advocate a holistic approach to consultation, which can benefit more than one student, Friend and Cook (1992) caution that it is unethical to give the impression that consultation will meet the needs of all the students in the class. This is especially true if the consultant's real agenda is to integrate students with special needs into the mainstream. Friend and Cook note that such an agenda undermines the idea of *shared* goals in consultation. Such goals are more likely to be shared if the teacher can be convinced that inclusion does benefit others in the class (Marks & Lewis, personal communication). Clarifying teachers' goals for the rest of the class and then indicating how participation in consultation could help the other students too may be a way of overcoming this resistance, but the consultant must be committed to those students as well.

In addition, if the consultee knows other teachers who have utilized consultation effectively, it can help. We have used our *It Works* newsletter (Figure 7.1) to advantage here because it lists techniques that other teachers have used to solve classroom problems. If the consultee agrees, a newsletter could publicize effective consultation approaches that have been utilized in that school.

A consultee may anticipate a high cost if *previous consultation experiences have been negative* (Meyers et al., 1979; Piersal, cited in Bergan, 1985). Here the consultant has the burden of proving that this time it will be different. Good listening skills (see Appendix A) are the first step, and teacher ownership of the consultation is critical. The consultant also needs to set limited goals before attempting

"IT WORKS"

What to Expect

The Child Study Team at Grant, Jefferson, and Wilson Schools are continually looking for ways to be helpful to the teachers and the staff we work with. By using this Newsletter. "It Works," teachers can see and learn from one another. The Newsletter will include descriptions of teaching techniques used in the classroom that the contributor feels work well with their students. Teachers can see what other teachers are doing well and can begin to use it themselves. Articles can describe any aspect of the classroom, including meaningful academic and behavioral strategies.

If you have contributed to the Newsletter and your article doesn't appear in the November edition, anticipate it will appear next month. Any teacher or staff member can contribute their ideas. Just complete a half of a page with your idea and give it to a Child Study Team member.

A PERSONAL TOUCH

Kindergarten—Wilson

As a Follow-through Kindergarten teacher, I know the importance of zeroing in on individual needs of children, diagnosing their strengths and weaknesses, and motivating them to meet daily goals through constant praise.

However, some children find it difficult to learn, in spite of ingenious teaching strategies. You have to give these children a "personal touch."

A hungry child will have difficulty learning. Maybe the school lunch is the only balanced meal this child receives. A sleepy child will have difficulty learning. Perhaps this child is not getting a proper amount of sleep each night. Children who are always an angry or disruptive have their reasons for behaving this way.

We have to take a personal look at each child. A good teacher will show concern by telling parents what he or she has observed in the classroom; ask parents questions about the child's home life; and give helpful suggestions. Teachers can refer parents to the school nurse, community agent, P.T.O., outside organizations, and of course, our Child Study Team. We cannot be good teachers and remain detached from our children.

STUDENT EVALUATIONS

Grade 2—Wilson

I have each child write an evaluation of me without having to sign their name. This gives the pupils a chance to let off steam and is also an insight as to how they feel about me. This is very helpful and enables me to make personal changes about myself and students. I encourage pupils to write exactly how they feel about me.

NAME OF CHANCE

Grade 3—Jefferson

Eliminate those familiar cries of "You always pick Susie" by using a name box: Print each child's name on a card and keep all names together in a decorated box. When an instant helper is needed, call upon the designated "keeper of the name box" to select a name at random. It works.

COMPLAINT BOX

Grade 6—Grant

I use a complaint box in my class. I take a shoe box and put a slit in the top. My students put any complaints in it that they feel should be brought to my attention. I used this first for disruptive pupils. Later I discovered that many of my shy pupils really felt secure using the box. Students may sign their names if they want to. They may also write if it is a group concern or for my eyes only. Sometimes the greatest asset of the box is that it enables pupils to let off steam without getting into trouble.

LUNCHROOM BEHAVIOR IMPROVEMENT PLAN

Assistant Principal—Grant

A behavior improvement plan is being used in our school cafeteria during lunch periods. Class(es) that demonstrate acceptable lunchroom behavior will receive a star for the particular lunch period. At the end of the month the classroom(s) with the largest total number of stars will receive a special bonus prize. The purpose of the stars and special bonus prize is to reinforce adherence to lunchroom rules. It is recommended that teachers continue to reinforce lunchroom rules in the classroom.

FIGURE 7.1. Staff newsletter.

holistic, system-oriented consulting. If the faculty is cynical about a workshop, the consultant should find out about past workshops and what went wrong (Schmuck, 1990). One such workshop in our district was ridiculed by teachers because it moralized and tried to create a "rah-rah" attitude toward improvement of teaching while offering little substantive help. Another such workshop failed because it dealt with general teacher stress rather than specific stressors within the school that needed to be changed. The alert consultant should digest this and develop a more relevant inservice to achieve consulting goals. Taking a look at meeting procedures is also relevant here (Schmuck, 1990) because if such procedures have been ineffective (disorganized and lacking teacher input into the agenda or into the actual meeting session), the meeting may go awry.

Also, *a treatment must be considered acceptable to the teacher* if the consultation method is to be implemented at all. Teachers prefer those interventions that are positive (Elliott, Witt, Galvin, & Peterson, 1984; Elliott, 1988) and require little time. If a proposed intervention is perceived to be practical, and makes sense to them, teachers are more likely to be willing to implement it (Whinnery, Fuchs, & Fuchs, 1991). Teachers knowledgeable about behavioral principles are more likely to view that type of treatment as acceptable (Skinner & Hales, 1992), but generally teachers prefer interventions described in humanistic, practical ways rather than in behavioral terminology (Witt, Moe, Gutkin, & Andrews, 1984). However, teachers who like an intervention will not necessarily feel it is feasible (Schumm & Vaughn, 1991), and experienced teachers are generally less likely to find any treatment acceptable (Witt et al., 1984).

Another problem causing resistance is that the consultee often wants immediate rewards whereas consultation typically has delayed rewards, and a delay in rewards may be perceived as an increase in costs. System knowledge is helpful here because knowing who in the system controls the rewards and punishments can help the consultant facilitate consultation by bringing these rewards into the situation. Reward power is a kind of authority usually associated with administrators and supervisors who control salary, benefits, and the like. Again, the consultant must be careful not to be perceived as an administrative power, for that will destroy the collaborative nature of the consultation. As an example, a consultant who helps a consultee publish the results of a consultation effort may bring in system reward without appearing to have direct reward power.

Another source of resistance based on personal costs comes from norm violations (Parsons & Meyers, 1984). Here the program suggested by the consultant—such as eliminating cursing behavior by ignoring it—runs contrary to school norms, which in this case might be to punish such behavior immediately. If the consultee promotes such a norm-violating approach, he/she may incur costs in the form of administrative or parental disapproval or even wrath.

Role conflict is another cause of resistance (Parsons & Meyers, 1984). There is a cost when teachers feel in conflict. In *interrole* conflict, the consultee struggles between the roles of caregiver for the students in the class and help seeker from the consultant. *Intrarole* conflict is similar but might take place with an administrator who feels that to be an efficient, effective principal, he/she needs to utilize consultation. On the other hand, the principal does not want to appear incompetent by sharing problems with the consultant. Here again the cost–reward ratio must be considered, both in the exogenous and endogenous sense.

Exogenous (external) costs involve such things as committing to meeting times or filling out behavior checklists. Endogenous costs involve dealing with inadequacies within the consultee. Parsons and Meyers (1984) use exchange theory (Thibaut & Kelley, 1959), in which we understand what people will do by weighing relationships in which rewards outweigh costs. If the rewards outweigh the costs, the consultant will be sought out. The opposite will cause resistance. Therefore, the consultant must look carefully at costs and rewards when working with consultees both on a personal as well as a systemic level. This can be done concretely by filling out a sheet of paper divided into two columns, labeling one column "costs" and the other "rewards." Consultants should try to list as many items as possible to anticipate the consultee's cost–reward reactions before they begin to consult (Parsons & Meyers, 1984).

Piersal (cited in Bergan, 1985) discusses D'Zurilla and Goldfried's (1971) problem-solving approach to resistance. He suggests integrating problem-solving techniques with applied behavior analysis and principles of learning in analyzing the resistance. In other words, just as a consultant might use problem-solving behavioral consultation to help a teacher solve a classroom problem, the same principles could help the consultant overcome a principal's or teacher's resistance. Just as the consultant would gather data on the frequency of a student's out-of-seat behavior, the consultant could also gather data on various forms of consultee resistance. The consultant could then define the problem behaviorally and brainstorm possible interventions, choosing an intervention such as using "I" statements or generating alternatives with the team member or teacher. Ideally, consultants would evaluate their results by analyzing taped conversations for verbal content, but this is probably impractical with a team, teacher, or principal who shows significant resistance. Consultants could also look for patterns in resistance to them as a means of gaining insight into how they are perceived.

Another way in which Parsons and Meyers look at resistance on the individual level is in terms of a problem in the *relationship* between consultant and consultee. The consultant needs to be sure the consultee does not have to fear punishment or loss. This is similar to the cost–reward ratio. Parsons and Meyers discuss cooperative versus competitive styles of both consultant and consultee. The consultant cannot be competitive or coercive when meeting with a competitive consultee, as this would result in stalemate. Rather, the consultant should place him/herself in a "one-down" position to defuse the resistance. A one-down position allows the consultee the upper hand by providing support and an accurate reflection of feelings. The consultant here has the job of asking questions to elicit the consultee's concerns and to confront the consultee with some aspect of his/her behavior that is forming the resistance. Such resistance, according to Piersal (cited in Bergan, 1985) can come from the following:

1. *Ignorance of the consultation process.* Consultees may have a "fear of the unknown" (Parsons & Meyers, 1984, p. 108). This can be assuaged by spelling out clearly what is involved in terms of the steps and assumptions of consultation (Rosenfield, 1987). Suggestions should be made tentatively, and the consultant should be careful not to oversell consultation.

2. *Incongruent expectations between the consultant and consultee.* The tendency in many districts to remove children from the classroom to remediate their special needs has conveyed to regular teachers that this is the only way to provide them with adequate instruction (McKenzie, 1972). For example, the teacher might say, "We did that consultation stuff; now let's get that student evaluated and placed" (Rosenfield, 1987; see also Witt, 1986). This becomes a school regularity; hence, there is resistance to alternatives (Witt, 1986). In instructional consultation (Rosenfield, 1987), the responsibility for change is placed squarely on the teacher because the quality of instruction is the source of most students' classroom problems. Therefore, more time and patience are required, and teachers must feel cared for and given timely and regular consultation services, especially if they are resistant types. Such careful cultivation is required if the teachers are expected to persist with a difficult consultation task, especially if it focuses on their teaching methods. Teachers who have high effectiveness levels, and therefore more

confidence in their ability to resolve problems, often prefer to make the decisions when utilizing consultation (DeForest & Hughes, 1992).

3. *Secondary gain.* Piersal indicates that having classroom problems may be in some way reinforcing to teachers. Perhaps it produces pity from others, attention from the principal, and so on. Therefore, the teacher may not really want the problem solved. Such an attitude may reflect what Caplan (1970) called lack of objectivity, or a need for confidence or recognition from others. The consultant here needs to work on building self-esteem and professional pride. An increase in confidence and a greater sense of ownership can help such staff members develop the courage to explore changes and take risks to make them.

4. *Conflicts with educational values.* Some teachers and principals believe in students' learning for intrinsic rewards rather than the extrinsic rewards often found in behavior-oriented programs. While learning for the intrinsic joy of it is laudable, research indicates that many students require extrinsic rewards for specific learning behaviors. Believing only in the intrinsic reflects a lack of objectivity, and the consultant needs to confront the consultee with the discrepancy between his/her belief and how he/she actually behaves (most teachers use extrinsic rewards even without realizing it), as well as the actual research data as to how children learn. Instruction in principles of behavior modification and problem-solving behavioral consultation might help some staff members, whereas others might prefer the collaborative approach of Idol and West. Behavioral approaches are often thought of rather simplistically by those not familiar with their details. Many teachers to whom I have spoken would say that a behavioral approach is equivalent to a token economy. Staff who are more ecologically oriented (that is, who look at the broader classroom environment and curriculum, class groupings, and structure of assignments) may find with pleasant surprise that such consultation carefully looks at those ecological considerations (see Chapter 1 for further discussion).

5. *Lack of respect for the autonomy and professional competence of the consultee* (Caplan, cited by Erchul, 1991). Some consultees fear being evaluated by the consultant (Parsons & Meyers, 1984). One way to show the consultee respect is to approach teachers from the perspective of *their* attitudes and values (Witt & Elliott, 1985) and talk about interventions using their own language (Rosenfield, 1987). Rosenfield stresses that the consultant must sense what life is like for the consultee.

In addition, the consultant must remember that the classroom is the teacher's sphere of influence, and most teachers do not like to have direct services provided in their classrooms (Speece & Mandell,

1980, cited by Gold & Hollander, 1992). Meyers's Level II approach to indirect service places more responsibility on the teacher, thereby easing territorial resistance.

6. *Admission of professional incompetence* (Caplan, 1970). Here the consultant needs to emphasize that rather than helping *consultees,* the task of consultation is to deal with student cases which problems are complicated, or confusing (Caplan, 1970). Meyers's confrontational techniques (Parsons & Meyers, 1984) can also be useful in helping consultees evaluate the difference between perceived incompetence and what they would like to learn, as well as sincerely accepting them as worthwhile human beings who have a right to express themselves and also a right to be less than fully knowledgeable in their field. Even a basic skill such as brainstorming may be something with which a teacher or administrator is not familiar, yet such skills are necessary for effective collaboration (Friend & Cook, 1992). Continued objections to classroom observation by consultants can be accommodated by having students learn self-monitoring or encouraging teachers to review tapes of their work by themselves.

7. *Seeing the consultant as a spy, having ax to grind, or as an unrealistic idealist* (Caplan, 1970). Consultants can deal with these views by raising questions that deepen their talks with teachers rather than trying to promote their expertise or trying to make changes. It is better to encourage the teacher to expand on his/her feelings, even if they are hostile. Even when the consultant becomes accepted, the mutual exploratory role definition and relationship building must be worked at as new people become the consultees. Teacher anxiety is often high during consultation (Kratochwill & Van Someren, 1985), and the consultant must be frequently present not only to model behavior, but to provide concern and warmth.

8. *Distorted perceptions.* This problem can be dealt with at staff meetings (Caplan, 1970; Sarason, 1982). For example, Meyers et al. (1979), when meeting with faculty and administrators, clearly spelled out through speeches and memos one key distorted perception of school psychologists as testers. Seeing the consultant as a tester and not as someone who regularly comes to work with and support teachers is a distortion that will cause resistance to attempts to consult.

EXTERNAL FACTORS IN RESISTANCE

Resistance often occurs when an organization or its individuals are mandated to change by forces beyond their control. This often occurs when legislation is passed, state or district regulations are imposed, or pressures are brought to bear to conform to national initiatives. Some potential pressures of this sort include the regular education initiative (Hallahan et al., 1988; Stemmel, Abernathy, Butera, & Lesar, 1991), the movement toward inclusion (Forest, 1988; Kune, n.d.), mentoring (Calliari, 1992), outcome-based education (Cobb, 1992; Elliott, 1992), and site-based management (Casey, 1992). All these programs will be coming, if they are not already in place, and schools will have to deal with the many changes required by these initiatives. (In this regard, reactive-type schools will have the most difficulty.) The consultant who wishes to achieve entry must prepare schools for such initiatives.

The regular education initiative (Hallahan et al., 1988) requires that mildly handicapped students be handled in regular classrooms. The inclusion movement goes even further, demanding that even the most severely and profoundly handicapped (the term "challenged" is preferable) children be given the opportunity for a socialization experience with "normal" children. It is postulated that so-called normal children will gain by being opened up to a more realistic view of these challenged people, seeing them as real people rather than as some distant oddity (H. Marks & Lynn Dee Lewis, personal communication, December 12, 1992). We can immediately see the resistance such an approach could create in anticipation of the great changes that would be required in personal values, classroom adaptations, and school policies (Smelter, Bradley, & Yudewitz, 1994). As Sarason (1982) has noted, schools do not take lightly to change. If a school district regularity includes the assumption that severely challenged people be isolated, there will be resistance to change at both organizational and individual staff levels. Those consultants who actually work in schools also know that there is resistance to accepting even mildly handicapped children in regular classes, particularly in view of schools' needs to be orderly and in control and to improve achievement test scores.

The move toward mentoring fosters resistance as well. One reason is that to mentor is to become a "broker" (Calliari, 1992). Here, the experienced teacher who is helping the new teacher adjust is guiding the new teacher toward resources. Resources include other teachers who, for example, could provide demonstration lessons within or outside the school. This involves crossing boundaries, which often creates resistance. The resistance could come from the other teachers, whose time is being imposed upon or whose skills are being exposed, or from administrators who see teachers mentoring other teachers as a threat to their supervisory prerogatives.

Outcome-based education seeks mastery of knowledge and skills essential to society's demands for students to be able to think critically, invent, solve problems, and continue to learn throughout their lifetime (Cobb, 1992). Graduation standards are changed from course credits or hour requirements to a mastery standard, which is measured through portfolios, demonstrations, products, and other evidence of specific skill mastery, often called authentic assessment (Elliott, 1992). Standardized normative testing, student tracking, and classifying of students would all be eliminated, according to Cobb (1992). Such changes in school regularities would require massive school curricular and attitude change, a real challenge for the consultant.

Site-based management (Casey, 1992), in which teachers have more of a voice in what happens in their school's policies, curriculum, discipline management, and so on, is a democratic philosophy that runs contrary to the bureaucratic (rigid, procedure-oriented) or autocratic nature of some schools. Casey (1992) cites a Rand study of site-based management that found that when such an approach is tried at an individual school, it becomes a reform of the entire *system*. It requires rethinking how schools are accountable, and it thrusts the parent into a key role for determining accountability. Hence, it would involve major changes in administrative prerogatives, greater responsibility for decision making by teachers who have not been used to it, and an increased voice by parents, who are not trained to help run schools.

Another external factor creating resistance is the requirement in many states that consultation be carried out before a child is classified (Harris & Cancelli, 1991). This places an implicit obligation on the teacher to consult, and on the administrator or principal to accept consultation. Consultation then loses its collaborative, voluntary nature, and resistance to its imposition may be generated.

HOW DOES RESISTANCE MANIFEST ITSELF?

Friend and Bauwens (1988) list six manifestations of resistance to consultation.

The Block

Sometimes the consultee just does not want to be involved. Although a collaborative orientation suggests that consultation not be done with such a person, the consultant should not give up at the first sign of resistance. The consultant needs to draw out the consultee to find out more about where the consultee stands, what the consultee wants, and what his/her concerns are. Strategies range from "I" statements and generating alternatives to clarifying what services are available. "I" statements are those that begin with the pronoun "I" and that share what the consultant feels is important. They do not attack the resistant consultee (see Appendix A for elaboration). At this early stage of resistance, it is better to find out more about the consultee's goals and values. It may also be important to clarify the nature of the adminis-trative sanction that exists. This is particularly important if the consultee is a principal and sanction initially came from the higher administration. While this might be construed as exercising "legitimate power" (Parsons & Meyers, 1984), the purpose is only to get a foot in the door.

As noted in Chapter 2, if the principal does not own the project, it will not work. Hence, when blocked by a principal, the consultant needs to reduce the desire for blockage by appealing to the principal's needs. Tying the consultation effort to those needs is one way to begin breaking through.

When being blocked by a teacher, it is better to back off and work with other teachers. Such resistance tends to break down when staff see their peers benefiting from the consultation. However, a careful analysis of the cost–benefit ratio for the resistant teacher may yield valuable information about why the block is being used.

The Stall

Often the consultee appears to accept the intervention but delays implementing it. For example, following a problem identification interview, the teacher agrees to gather some observational data on a student's out-of-seat behavior. At the next meeting, the teacher tells the consultant that there was no time because of demands to mark papers, to attend a school committee meeting, and so on. Here consultants must ask themselves whether their approach has been truly collaborative. Perhaps in an attempt to be agreeable, the teacher took on more of a burden than planned, and in reality did not want to take time from the lesson plan to record these data. The consultant should find out why this was not communicated, try an alternative that requires a minimum of time to implement, and specify in writing who is to do each task and when each should complete it. Our Consultation Progress Report (see Chapter 3, Figure 3.2) is one way of accomplishing this task. The teacher may need to be drawn into the process and convinced that data gathering is a worthwhile time investment. Therefore, the consultant should gather the data in the hope that the consultee will see the value once the data are available.

The Reverse

Here the consultee is verbally positive but rather than delaying, as in the stall, does not follow through ever. Once again, the responsibilities probably have not been spelled out clearly enough or the consultee does not own the process sufficiently. The teacher must be included in all aspects of the planning, and feedback must be obtained frequently. Confrontation (Meyers et al., 1979; Gross, 1980, cited by Wickstrom & Witt, 1993) may be necessary in this situation, but it should be done in a positive, empathic way that presents the consultee with the contradiction between what was agreed to and what was actually done. One reason for the confrontation is to help the consultee acknowledge that at least part of him/her does not want to do this, perhaps by saying, "Sometimes when a new approach is used, a part of us really is anxious to try it, but another part is pretty skeptical. Do you think that might apply to you?" Such willingness to hear the other side of the story may itself be enough to dissolve the resistance. At the very least, the confrontation can help the consultant find out what was left unsaid or unclarified when the initial consultation was done. Hence, the consultee is made "aware" that there is a contradiction and then helped to develop strategies to overcome the conflict (Meyers et al., 1979).

The Projected Threat

In this situation, the teacher fears that the principal will not like what is being done. The teacher may have doubts as to the acceptability of certain interventions or may be skeptical of consulting in general. Gutkin and Bossard (1984) found that teachers whose principals encouraged their autonomy were more likely to prefer consultation to referring students for evaluation. Wickstrom and Witt (1993) discuss how important issues of freedom are to teachers. The strategy recommended by Friend and Bauwens (1988) is to get the principal to specify support for the consultation effort. It is quite important to be sure that such sanction exists before meeting with individual teachers. A memo from the principal to teachers, perhaps via a newsletter announcement about the consultant's availability in the building, is helpful. Of course, an open meeting at which the consultant speaks to the faculty, after being introduced by the principal, is another way of demonstrating such sanction.

The Guilt Trip

Using this technique, the consultee tries to make the consultant feel guilty for making the consultee suffer through consultation. Such suffering may be caused by having to put up with a difficult student longer or by having to teach one student skills that the rest of the class has mastered. The consultant can deal with this by minimizing demands on the consultee, respecting time constraints, and asking for alternative suggestions. Showing the teacher how other students could benefit (e.g., by participating in peer tutoring of the identified client) could ease the burden (see Maheady, Harper, Mallette, & Winstanley, 1991). Often, data I have gathered on disruptive students showed that the percentage of time spent in disruption was much less than the teacher estimated. Such data could help lessen the guilt the teacher may place on the consultant.

Consultants also need to look at how they handle guilt. If they are easily made to feel guilty, it would help to more closely examine themselves and try to increase their ability to look at a situation objectively. Rational–emotive and cognitive therapies specify that internal beliefs and thought processes, not accusations from others, are the causes of internal guilt (Ellis, 1962). If the consultant is prone to think that because someone says something bad about him/her it is probably true, and that he/she ought to be ashamed for, for example, harassing this overburdened teacher, it will be very hard for the consultant to help that teacher. The consultant needs to ask what makes it true (e.g., Is he/she really harassing the consultee?), and what proof he/she has that he/she should feel shameful and guilty about it, regardless of whether the consultee is readily feeling pressure. Focusing on the objective nature of the problem identification process can also help solve the problem, for example: "Yes, I can see that you are feeling much pressure from our working with instead of removing this student, but if we can reduce the frequency and intensity of the oppositional behavior, that pressure could be eased significantly." This is a problem-solving rather than a self-blaming approach.

Tradition

"We've always done it this way." Friend and Bauwens (1988) suggest that this statement reflects a need for safety (Maslow, 1954). It may also suggest a need to identify with the school's culture and regularities (Maslow's belongingness need). When a consultee has such a strong need, the consultant must use support and praise. The method of intervention should be compatible with the teacher's style, so that it will not be seen as a major change. If a teacher's style is somewhat directive and authoritative, a problem in classroom management might be addressed through an approach such as assertive discipline (Canter, 1989). This method combines positive reinforcement with a focus on a graded series of negative consequences for clearly specified disruptive behavior. It reinforces teacher authority by demanding such behavior as hand raising before students verbalize anything. The consultant must also be aware of school culture issues so that he/she can counter any perceptions of conflicts with the culture.

VOLUNTARISM AS AN ISSUE IN RESISTANCE

A key issue for the consultee is willingness to participate in consultation. Gutkin and Curtis (1990) assert that there is no certainty that teachers are predisposed to be active participants in consultation. Harris and Cancelli (1991) have questioned whether collaborative consultation really is truly collaborative. They examined "volunteerism" (sic) in teachers, noting that true voluntary involvement in consultation results in a greater consultee investment in it. If voluntarism is so important, how does this reconcile with consultant power?

I have discussed how consultants can use their expert and referent power to aid in entry. Harris and Cancelli (1991) stressed that consultants often also have other forms of power available to them, which French and Raven (1959) attribute to those who have *line authority*. These could include reward power, coercive power, and legitimate power. Those who possess reward power control the purse strings and privileges available to teachers. Coercive power belongs to those who can make people do things, and legitimate power is obtained via election or appointment as leader. Because consultants can often obtain rewards for teachers such as course credits (reward power), make teachers do consultation because a principal mandates it (coercive power), or be a gatekeeper to special education (legitimate power, because many consultants are assigned to do just that), they then possess powers *that run contrary to any form of voluntarism,* which is essential to true collaborative consulting. The consultant could also be elected to head a student assistance committee and face the same dilemma.

Harris and Cancelli also caution that the use of expert power may also run contrary to true voluntarism, because true collaboration defines the teacher–consultee as an expert too (Pugach & Johnson, 1989). The consultant who wishes to be effective must respect the other's expert power, especially since the teacher has the real power in many instances to make the consultation a success or failure.

Harris and Cancelli (1991) assert that most of us do not assess the willingness of the consultee to enter into the consultation, though this is considered a critical element in the collaborative consultation competencies listed by West and Cannon (1988). One can measure levels of consultee willingness at time of entry, during problem identification, and at the intervention and follow-up stages of consultation. The Teacher Involvement Scale (DeForest & Hughes, 1992) can be used to measure degree of involvement at the three stages of problem identification, problem assessment, and intervention planning.

A consultee who volunteers for consultation may have various levels of commitment to the process. At entry, for example, the consultation could be teacher initiated, consultant initiated, or even mandated by supervisors. A teacher may not let the consultant know that the mandate was there, but it will affect the voluntary nature of the response. Even if a consultee has been willing to participate from beginning to end, the consultant may be resistant to pursuing alternative interventions after the plan has been implemented and evaluated.

Harris and Cancelli (1991) suggest that the consultant use referent power to help the teacher become comfortable with the process, to be sure there are no pressures operating to defeat true voluntarism, to maximize consultee choices, and to try to get the consultee to generate some *effort*. Effort seems to create investment in the process; so does level of participation when employees are faced with changes in job role expectations (Coch & French, 1948). Effort can mean spending time in the library learning new information or in the classroom collecting data. The consultant's strategy is to help teachers feel an ownership of the process and encourage them to discuss the negatives as well as the positives of consultation.

CONSULTANT ISSUES IN RESISTANCE

Self-Awareness

Special services team members or outside consultants must do careful self-analysis to understand how their own issues generate resistance to the consultation and affect their willingness to push themselves to do consultation.

One such issue is the *need to build motivation to solve problems.* The inside consultant may feel the pressure of having to serve other schools or teachers, or may be behind on mandated reevaluation tasks. The outside consultant may have teaching pressures or demands from other research and writing projects which make it difficult to spend the necessary time in the schools to build relationships and reduce resistance. As noted earlier, it takes much time to work with staff to identify problems, gather data, and work on interventions. The motivation to problem-solve can be encouraged by effective time scheduling (see Chapter 8), so that the consultant is sure other demands are being met while he/she invests time in the specified consultation project.

A careful examination of a consultant's own needs will also shed light on any hesitance to immerse him/herself in the consulting process. The consultant can use the Maslow (1954) needs hierarchy to see which needs (e.g., safety, belongingness, esteem, or self-actualization) are behind his/her desire to consult. Evaluating the benefits (and costs) accruing to the consultant may help increase his/her motivation. Benefits could include increased staff regard (esteem), camaraderie (belongingness), improved knowledge and skill, and a general sense of growth (esteem and self-actualization). The latter comes from a desire to stretch oneself beyond the usual task demands (e.g., evaluations or counseling). If an inside consultant is more comfortable with a predictable work assignment, he/she may want to reconsider doing consultation. Consultation is not for everyone. Particularly for the conventional personality type of consultant (Holland, 1966), who values routine and prefers to avoid conflict or the pressures of assertion, consultation will not be a comfortable role. However, the consultant's concern for detail may be useful in helping other members of the team with data gathering and analysis.

The consultant's own self-awareness is therefore quite important. Consultants cannot separate their own orientation from their behavior in the consulting situation. They must be aware of their own dynamics and needs and be sure that those needs have been adequately cared for (Fine et al., 1979) if they are to be effective helpers to others. Fine, Grantham, and Wright note that too close an identification with the problems of the consultee will reduce the consultant's ability to be a true facilitator. Consultants cannot be rescuers if their goal is to consult.

Involving Coworkers

Special services staff may face paranoia from other team or special services staff members. These others fear that a consulting staff member will gain more status or have an easier job than doing continuous evaluations (Newman, 1967). Such issues can be dealt with in team and department meetings, and often involve the team-building techniques discussed in Chapter 3. Such concerns were quite prevalent among other special services teams not involved in my consultation project. Sharing information, asking for input from them, and helping them see the heavy load the consultants were carrying helped to ease their suspicion.

The consultant needs a peer support network (Conoley & Conoley, 1982) for help in evaluating ethical dilemmas and simply providing feedback and assistance with the many difficulties of consulting. If a consultant's own team does not provide this help, the consultant should seek out others in the school or university environs. However, consultants should not neglect the opportunity to do greater team building, so that such support may be forthcoming from their own group (see Chapter 3 for elaboration).

Not Going It Alone

The consultant cannot be the sole resource for the consultee or his/her effectiveness will be reduced. There is a sense of aloneness and of being overwhelmed that comes from allowing oneself to be put in that position (Fine et al., 1979). However, it can be tempting to be the only one depended on. Such a situation can feed the consultant's need to be omnipotent (Ellis, 1962), a kind of "being everything to everyone" syndrome. This is related to Maslow's (1954) esteem need and is connected with the desire for power over others, a rather negative means of achieving esteem.

Being Objective with Coworkers

Fine et al. (1979) also emphasize the need for the *inside* consultant to develop a contract to minimize resistance. Although the special services staff member within the system is often expected to be available to teachers and give advice, this expectation may be quite different from what the consultant is willing or able to do, and so those services should be spelled out explicitly. It may not be easy for a consultant who has known a teacher or principal quite well to sit down and specify or negotiate exactly what commitments will be made, but it is quite important to defuse resistance based on misperceptions of the process.

Being Too Authoritarian

Many professionals do not realize the importance of consultation being *consultee*-centered (Erchul, 1991, interviewing Caplan). They are more authoritarian or procedure-oriented in their work, and may lean toward an advice-giving role, neglecting to create ownership of the consulting with the consultee. Such professionals should try to become aware of the benefits of the collaborative method. Their resistance may reflect a need to build self-confidence. It takes confidence on the part of the consultant to allow others to share ownership of classroom problem solving.

Authoritarian attitudes, along with other dysfunctional approaches, can sabotage the consultant. Conoley and Conoley (1982) cite Rae-Grant's work on how consultants fail. With minor variations, some of these approaches include:

1. Ignoring the norms of the organization: using telephones without asking, being late and unreliable, and dressing anyway you like.
2. Talking with one consultee about another or reporting to administrators about staff behaviors.
3. Waiting in the office to be approached for service.
4. Criticizing the system whenever possible.
5. Failing to build a relationship with the top administrator.
6. Appearing aloof and formal. (Instead of asking questions about the consultee's life, the consultant spends time talking about his/her own life and accomplishments and learns nothing about the consultee.)
7. Being dependent on administrator support and having frequent meetings with top administrators to structure every activity.
8. Announcing the intention to engage in activities that fit the consultant's *own* interests and agendas. (This amounts to conspiring to cause unwanted and unsanctioned change. Being unaware of motives is a trap and a guarantee to build resistance in others.)

Conoley and Conoley (1982) cite additional ways a consultant might fail, also based on Rae-Grant's writings. These include being an unyielding know-it-all, sulking when advice is not taken (instead of using it as a valuable feedback experience), keeping professional status too much in the forefront, forming alliances with subgroups, picking a few consultees to be therapy patients, and interpreting the consultee's motives using all available jargon. Most of these behaviors involve being self- rather than other-centered and reflect a failure to tune in to the consultee. Some of the suggestions in Appendix A may help here but cannot make for basic personality change if consultants have no empathic awareness of others and of the system in which they work.

Consultants exhibit many of the same characteristics often seen in consultees. One important similarity is staff inertia or momentum in an anticonsulting direction (Newman, 1967; Gresham, 1991). Consultant resistance often occurs in an attempt to maintain the status quo and when consulting teachers or special services teams suffer burnout from being stretched too thin already (Friend & Bauwens, 1988). Gresham noted that factors such as frequency and intensity of treatments and their acceptability are often ignored by people who want to change student behavior. Such factors also must be considered by the consultant wishing to change *staff* behavior. Here the consultant must look at how often to intervene or to be available to school staff for consultation, and how intense the effort is.

Another factor accounting for a consultant's own resistance to doing consulting is lack of training (Dyck & Dettmer, 1989). Many consultants are not trained to analyze the verbalizations of the consulting session precisely, to properly utilize problem identification skills, to role-play, to model, to reinforce, and to give proper feedback (Kratochwill & Van Someren, 1985). A consultant whose skills are weak in any of these areas can look for further training in the key texts in the consultation field, additional formal course work, or help from colleagues. (See Kratochwill & Bergan, 1990, and West, Idol, & Cannon, 1989, for two good texts with accompanying workbooks.)

A FRAMEWORK FOR ENTRY

Maher and colleagues (Maher & Bennett, 1984) developed the DURABLE framework for the implementation of consultation. I believe, as do others (Ponti et al., 1988), that the DURABLE approach may help achieve effective entry, minimize resistance to consultation, and provide a conceptual framework if used with the four targeted levels of Parsons and Meyers (1984). In addition, this structure helps in evaluating whether consultation has been successful and why. The DURABLE approach provides a structure to check how the consultant handles each step of consulting. It includes adaptations by Ponti et al. (1988) and myself. Such an approach can be utilized at Meyers's Levels II, III and IV. The structure is as follows:

Discussing: The consultant clarifies the goals of helping more students and teachers in a timely manner. The goal of reducing special education referrals is discussed, as are practical Level IV issues such as staff involvement, recordkeeping, meeting schedules, and so on. At Level II—the level of indirect service to the client—resistance can be reduced by discussing concerns about reducing referrals to special education.

Understanding: Here the consultant tries to increase the school's understanding (Level IV) of why consultation is necessary at this time and to deal with such concerns as less funding or staff layoffs if fewer referrals are made to special education. Making sure that teachers have an understanding of how consultation can help them cope with the identified client is a Level II intervention.

Reinforcing: The consultant reinforces staff efforts to expand roles to do more consulting (Level III) and tries to obtain reinforcement for staff participation by providing release time (Level IV). Finding ways to reinforce teachers for their efforts in gathering objective information is a Level II effort.

Adapting: The consultant tries to adapt school policy to encourage interventions prior to referral for assessment and to change job descriptions of special services teams to include consultative functions (Level IV), while encouraging teachers to grow (Level III) through making adaptations in role and function that include serving a broader range of students.

Building: The consultant tries to build up efficacy expectations of the staff by emphasizing the success others have had with consultative efforts (Level III). Commitment is also built to make changes by involving school staff (Levels III and IV). Building teacher esteem and efficacy is a Level III intervention.

Learning: This step includes inservice training for staff in consultation and teaming strategies so they can participate effectively in the prereferral process (Levels III and IV). Learning about the teacher's need for further training in such skills as brainstorming (Friend & Cook, 1992), if they are to be more effective at problem definition and finding interventions, is a Level III intervention. Learning also takes place on the part of the consultant (e.g., that teachers are often inconvenienced if the inservice training takes place in the hours before or after school).

Evaluating: Helping teachers to see how evaluating intervention data can be critical in developing efficacy. In a successful consultation program, one must evaluate whether most of the staff used the consultation assistance; whether requests for consultation increased;

whether special services staff roles actually changed; and whether there were changes in student, teacher, and administrator behavior.

SUMMARY

Resistance can be reduced by obtaining administrative support; actively involving teachers from the start; creating benefits such as team teaching opportunities as rewards for teachers who participate; gathering data on the effectiveness of consultation, so that teachers and principals can see that it works; and making the intervention fit the values of the teachers. In addition, consultants should highlight novelty, respect turf, give nonjudgmental feedback, work on developing a trusting relationship, and develop consultation slowly but consistently (Friend & Bauwens, 1988). If consultation does not appear to work and resistance appears, the consultant must backtrack through the consultation stages to identify what went wrong and where to make changes. The consultant also must be willing to look inward yet cannot neglect external pressures on the system, which might generate resistance.

Much resistance comes from the consultant's not being attuned to the school culture, climate, or teachers' and principals' feelings and attitudes. If the consultant obtains sufficient training to be comfortable with skills ranging from reflective to behavior-analysis techniques, from modeling and role play to brainstorming and objective observation, resistance will become much less of an issue. The consultant needs to form a basic acceptance of the school as a culture in its own right and realize that change in any school is often a slow, tedious process in which small steps are taken to recognize staff needs and develop alliances with administrators and teachers.

8

Handling Logistics

Aside from issues of resistance, there are other blocks to successful consulting. This chapter attempts to help the special services staff member and consultant with practical, logistical steps to make consultation entry easier.

To aid the consultant's effectiveness, sometimes simple, even obvious, measures must be taken. I never cease to be amazed how both inside and outside consultants and regularly employed special services personnel get so absorbed in their day-to-day duties that they neglect to use the aids and services in a school that can make their job easier.

I have found that investing some time at the beginning of a school year to obtain information on how the school schedules students and teachers, where report cards and district scores can be located, and how to find out about students' attendance and cutting patterns pays off in efficiency throughout the year. It is also wise for the consultant to be prepared for schoolwide events that may interfere with his/her consultation, and to know how to make the best use of such interruptions. In this chapter I provide suggestions for handling these types of questions.

FINDING PEOPLE

The consultant or special services personnel, who is very likely to be itinerant, cannot function without being able to see teachers during the times that he/she is in the school. I have seen consultants try to accomplish this task without any of the materials available to them from the various school offices. Carrying a file of the following items is a requirement for the effective consultant or special services team member.

1. *Teacher schedules.* Teacher schedules should list exactly where a teacher is each period of the school day, including the room number, subject taught, lunch time, and free periods. If the consultant wants to observe a class or have a conference, this schedule will tell him/her when it is possible. Often a consultant comes into a school and expects to be able to meet with staff at his/her convenience. This is both unrealistic and inconsiderate.

When looking for a teacher's free periods on a schedule, the consultant cannot always assume that the teacher is willing to give up a preparatory period or a lunch to meet with the consultant. However, having a schedule in hand when talking with a teacher makes it easier to adjust and set up alternative meeting times.

2. *Department schedules.* These schedules help the consultant see at a glance when more than one teacher is free. Often the consultant needs to meet with an entire department. If all staff members are not free at the same time, there may at least be groups with which one could meet.

Schedules of "specials" (when students are at gym, art, basic skills, or other special subject areas) are also very helpful in finding students and teachers, and in connecting with these staff members. Such schedules are especially helpful at the elementary school level. When an elementary class is at art or gym, the academic teacher is often available for consultation.

3. *Grade schedules.* These schedules give the consultant an idea where groups of teachers and students are, because they are listed by grade, section, and availability. Holistic consultation encourages the consultant to work with groups of same-grade teachers, or whole classes, and such schedules make that possible.

4. *Student schedules.* These schedules are available from the students themselves or can be obtained from the main office or the central computer. In some districts, such schedules are not made readily available to consultants, but if they are the consultant should be sure to know which vice principal or administrator handles them.

Schedules are needed for elementary students because many are taken out of class for basic skills (Title I) tutoring and minor subjects. Schedules are even more essential in tracking junior high and high school students or any students on departmentalized schedules. If the consultant is evaluating such students, he/she should know when they have lunch to plan the length of testing. Starting an evaluation at 11:00 A.M. and belatedly discovering the student has lunch at 11:30

will interrupt the process and may require the consultant to return at another time.

Schedules show consultants the balance between regular education and special education courses, so they have a sense of the demands on a student. Schedules make observation in varied settings possible, because the consultant can choose an academic subject, gym, or a vocational/hands-on minor subject. Schedules also help the consultant understand the pressures a student faces. A learning disabled student with five class periods before lunch may have more than he/she can handle. Scheduling a student with an attention deficit disorder for study halls and other unstructured time may be inviting trouble. A student passing four courses and failing three may have the failing subjects the last three periods. This tells the consultant that the student may be cutting class and leaving school early because of a problem, or may simply be fatigued by the end of the day. The consultant who is aware of these contingencies can work with the counselor or scheduling staff to find a better balance.

5. *Course schedules.* Irregular course schedules and changes in course locations can present quite a challenge to the consultant. For example, just as I thought I had mastered all the intricacies of a large high school's scheduling, I went to meet with a student in the vocational–technical school attached to our high school. It was during the second report period of an exploratory program. In the exploratory program, our students rotate through four shops throughout the school year. Only the first shop was listed on the district's computer and now the student was in a different shop. The vice principal in charge of the vocational–technical school had a schedule showing which students rotate to which shops and in what order. If I had not known where to go to find such a schedule, it would have been almost impossible to find this student.

6. *Bell schedules.* In a large secondary school, bell schedules are critical for knowing when each period begins and ends. Many schools have varied bell schedules, depending on the program for the day. If there is a long assembly or homeroom or a half-day inservice for teachers, the bell schedule changes. Sometimes even the sequence of class periods is reversed or altered. Unwary consultants can waste a trip to the school if students and teachers they expect to see are not available at that time, or if the periods in which they planned to see the teacher or student are shortened.

7. *Field trip schedules.* Sometimes students and teachers are unavailable because they have gone on field trip. Often the consultant needs some of the other schedules we have discussed to know who has gone on a trip. For example, a trip may be organized on the basis of

homeroom or subject. Knowing that a student has been on such a trip can give the consultant an opening for rapport building in later conversations with the student. Moreover, consultants who can free themselves up to go along on such a trip have an excellent opportunity to get to know students and teachers in a different setting.

8. *Finding absent students.* As noted in Chapter 5, it is important to cultivate a relationship with the attendance staff. Consultants cannot deal with students who are not in school. Attendance or absence lists are collected by many schools. Sometimes these lists are available in the homerooms, where attendance is taken. At small schools, the main office usually has the information. At larger schools, consultants will have to look at the central computer data to obtain this information. Many schools print out a list of who is absent that day, which is usually made available to inside staff, but outside consultants may have to search for such lists. Here again, the relationship with other staff, including secretaries, can be critical if the consultant needs such information. Attendance staff often have sanction to go to the homes of students or to track down students in the neighborhood. They telephone parents, and often have emergency numbers to reach parents. They may even be able to bring in parents who have no transportation.

The best way to obtain all the above schedules and lists is through the school's main office. The consultant may be able to do this easily and quickly through the secretaries, or he/she may have to approach vice principals, department heads, or principals for sanction to obtain such information. Some larger schools have special attendance or computer departments that make scheduling information available.

PASSES

Many schools require passes for students and visitors. The itinerant special services team member or consultant is often considered a "visitor" rather than a school employee. Thus, consultants must often sign in and out and obtain a pass to move around the building. Consultants must have some identification, along with a pass, when they go to get a student. When the student leaves the consultant, he/she may need a pass to go back to class. The consultant's identification can also have public relations value, as a kind of introduction to strangers on the staff.

The need for passes raises a deeper issue of the sanction required to see various people throughout the school. (This issue is also discussed in Chapter 2.) Many principals and other administrators, in an attempt to control their schools, limit who a consultant can see, at least until the consultant becomes trusted (Conoley & Conoley, 1982). Conoley and Conoley stress how important it is to respect these limits if the consultant is to build trust. My own experience as an inside consultant is that eventually I have been granted freedom to see anyone in a given school, but only after having carefully built trust by abiding by the school's rules and restrictions, no matter how unreasonable (see Chapter 2 for elaboration).

MEETING ROOMS

Many schools use every room they can find. Funded programs such as special education, bilingual education, basic skills (Title I tutoring), and grant programs each require school rooms regardless of how small their enrollments. The consultant is often given low priority in terms of room privileges. Sometimes using class schedules is the simplest way for the consultant to determine when a room is free. Secretaries and maintenance people usually know when rooms are open, and will give the consultant keys if he/she treats them with respect. A list of teachers absent for the day may provide a clue to an available room, if no substitute teacher has come in. Field trips also free up rooms.

Rooms to consider include school libraries, when the librarian is at lunch; teacher lunchrooms and lounges when lunch is over, or at times when no free periods are scheduled; counselor's, nurse's, and special program offices; and music, art, and vocational rooms when those staff are at lunch. Consultants may have to get used to using book storage rooms, the main lunchroom during nonlunch periods, or even gym rooms or offices. Secretaries may let the consultant use their desks when they are absent or at lunch, and even janitorial rooms can be satisfactory for meetings. If consulting with teachers, their classroom is often the best place, because they may have student records and work to which they will want to refer.

WHEN CONSULTEES AND STUDENTS
ARE UNAVAILABLE

Consultation at Levels I and II requires student observation. A schedule of special school events may help in finding them, if they are not in a scheduled class. School events in the auditorium, gym, or outside on a field sometimes provide unique opportunities for consultants to observe staff–student interaction. If the goal is student observation, the consultant must be cautious not to call attention to the student or to cause embarrassment. Sometimes a note to a staff member in charge of the event will produce an unobtrusive identification of the student. It is preferable for the consultant to meet with the student at a prearranged place rather than to walk out of a public place like an auditorium, or even classroom, with a student.

When visiting a school to see certain teachers or students, consultants should have alternative people on their list in the case of absences or the occurrence of special programs. (Carrying a schedule file saves valuable time in tracking down additional students or teachers.) Special auditorium programs for students often free teachers to talk to consultants. Student testing programs rarely involve all students, so consultants should see if anyone they need has been exempted. These can also be good times to talk to other school personnel (secretaries, maintenance people, etc.). Ideally, the consultant should turn "downtime" into networking opportunities. If no one is available, the consultant should have work to do that is desk-oriented. He/she can write or dictate reports, score classroom observations or tests, plan interventions, and so on, but only if he/she has planned for such contingencies.

SCHOOL GEOGRAPHY ISSUES

Elementary versus Junior High and High School

Wary consultants will tune in to the subtle and not-so-subtle differences when dealing at different school levels. In my experience, elementary schools are run more rigidly by their administrators, and elementary school teachers respond better to a rigid, structured environment than do upper-school personnel. For example, the rules are usually stricter regarding where teachers have to be at different times, as they are responsible for the same group of students for most of the day. Newman (1967) asserted that the heavy workload and the way that elementary teachers conceptualize leads to "compulsive obedience to authority" and little time to reflect on or experiment with new ways of doing things.

In junior high schools and especially high schools, there is typically more staff freedom consonant with the increasing freedom given to students, who are seen as young adults instead of children. However, in these settings, isolation becomes more of an issue (Newman, 1967).

The consultant's role here is to work on building professional self-awareness and self-esteem, whereas in the elementary setting, the consultant may emphasize helping teachers cope with sometimes rigid supervision. Of course, there is great variation among school settings, and consultants may have to reverse this emphasis depending on the needs of particular staff members.

Upper-school staff, because their certifications require them to be specialists, sometimes see themselves as better than the elementary school "superficial" generalist teachers (Sarason, 1982). Sarason notes that a greater number of male teachers at the secondary level also encourages the view that the secondary student is a budding young adult. Secondary teachers, regardless of sex, demand more responsibility and adult behavior from their students. On the other hand, the elementary school child has to be taken care of by the often female teacher, who is seen as a child-care specialist. This caring role does make elementary settings fertile ground for consultation entry. As the elementary teacher often knows his/her students better than does the secondary teacher, who may only see the student one period per day, he/she can provide more information. Also, because the elementary teacher is working with the same group most of the day, it is easier to gather data on instructional organization and strategies. There is a greater chance that changes made through consultation will be transferred to the identified student and class, because of the continued exposure to the same teacher. At junior high or high school, the departmental schedule means that the consultant has to meet with more teachers in order to effect consistent changes.

The special services staff member may be seen as more of an authority figure in the elementary setting. This can have both positive and negative implications. Elementary teachers may be more open to concrete consultant suggestions but may also expect a less equal relationship than current concepts of collaborative consultation warrant (Parsons & Meyers, 1984; Idol & West, 1987; Zins, 1992). The consultant who is put in an authority role in an elementary setting will also be saddled with the responsibility when interventions do not work. On the other hand, if the consultant acts like an authority in a junior high or high school, he/she may be ridiculed or perhaps politely ignored. I have observed that the culture of the latter settings fosters greater freedom from authoritative control.

At upper-school levels, teachers are more open and will demand parity with consultants. The consultant may have to work harder to gain their respect, and they will be more outspoken in their criticisms than elementary staff are. Elementary staff, if displeased with the consultant, are more likely to respond in a passive–aggressive manner, finding excuses not to apply the intervention or agreeing to it and then doing what they want. For instance, when I once told an elementary teacher (after an observation) that she gave no positive reinforcement to her class, she commented that she had not realized this and would do so in the future. She added that she could monitor her responses from here on in and did not need the consultant to observe whether increased reinforcement occurred or was helpful in class management. Although this teacher remained superficially friendly to me, I lost access to her class. In good collaborative consultation, this teacher would have looked over the observation data and formed her own conclusions, which she would then have acted on in ways that she and I developed. I made the mistake of becoming so excited about the clarity and implications of the observational data that I neglected the most important aspect of collaborative consultation: that of the teacher's role of participation and ownership.

Physical Environment

Other aspects of school geography include a sense of the physical environment and location of classrooms and departments. Some schools isolate their special education classes in certain sections of the building. This makes it easy for consultants to find special education staff and students, but also tells them how the department is perceived or perceives itself. Others group areas similarly (e.g., science and math). Knowing where departments are saves time for the consultant and also directs the consultant to the people he/she needs to get to know. Picking the right rooms for an activity also is important. A music or art room with all the distracting equipment would not be the best setting for counseling a group of hyperactive students (unless these activities were programmed into the group's agenda, and then, only with the OK of the teacher in that room).

Another school geography entry issue is locating where the teachers "hang out." Not all are in the faculty lunchroom or lounge. Some prefer the gym, where they can work out during free times. Some might go to a favorite neighborhood restaurant if they have time to leave the school. Some take walks. (A consultant can consult while taking a walk too.) Other teachers may prefer to be by themselves during free times yet are open to a call at home later. The flexible consultant knows where and when teachers prefer to meet.

SCHOOL EVENTS

Various school events and business also can get in the way of effective consulting.

Emergency Faculty Meetings

When emergency meetings are called, the consultant's schedule is again thrown off. However, this is another opportunity to observe the school culture, this time when it is in crisis. Consultants can observe who responds to the urgent issue and how: which faculty members are assertive and which are aggressive, which mumble to themselves and say nothing publicly. How does the principal handle a crisis? What kind of management style does he/she show? Sometimes the consultant can offer ideas to help the situation. The very nature of the crisis can propel the consultant from relative obscurity into significant recognition. If the emergency meeting concerns such issues as a discipline crisis, new pressure from evaluating bodies, or a sudden push to have all teachers observed, the consultant can offer constructive ideas and programs if he/she is systemically oriented.

The Fire Drill

During a fire drill, all people have to leave the school promptly. This is disruptive to classroom observations, evaluation, data gathering, counseling, and consulting. Nowadays, a fire "drill" is often the real thing and takes a long time. I have experienced school evacuations that lasted as long as 1 hour or more because of bomb threats. It is in the consultant's interest to have extra work to carry along. This can be a good time to plan a schedule for the coming days or to write up a consultation plan. The consultant could also utilize the time to observe students and teachers. Consultants may be asked to improve behavior during fire drills, and experiencing them firsthand is necessary to perform this service. Sometimes, quiet talk with teachers and other staff can take place; the consultant can get to know secretaries and aides and can again observe an administrator's style of leadership.

Preholiday Parties and Programs

Special events can throw off consultation efforts because they take students and teachers away. As simple an event as a Christmas party, a Thanksgiving play, or a spring concert can tie up students, teachers, administrators, and rooms. The consultant, by using the schedule file, can anticipate such events and try to make the best of them.

Student observation can be carried on during special assemblies and programs. Students often behave differently in such settings than they do in the academic one. For example, many special needs students shine when given opportunities in drama, music, or art. Some of these special program teachers may not even know that the student singing in their holiday festival is classified as a special needs student.

In addition to learning about students, the consultant can learn about effective and ineffective teacher styles by watching preparations for a play or how students are guided through an art project for a special event. Sometimes the usual discipline and formality ease during such events, and it is an opportunity for the consultant to blend in more easily. Sharing punch and cookies at a class party, for example, can go a long way toward effective entry. Parties can be used for assessment purposes as well, in terms of observing socialization patterns, doing sociograms, measuring adaptive skills (cooking, making invitations, baking, etc.) and academic survival skills (following recipes, doing practical math calculation), and assessing verbal development (memorizing and delivering parts in plays or musical selections) and visual–motor coordination (cutting, fingering musical instruments, centering artwork, printing, decorating, drawing).

WHO CAN PROVIDE WHICH SERVICES TO WHOM?

Getting around the designated funding dilemma can be quite a problem. The consultant often runs into difficulty crossing federal funding lines in such areas as bilingual education and basic skills or remedial education (Title I), as well as special education, where the special services teams so often function. For example, I created a problem when I recommended, without going through proper channels, that a student be removed from a basic skills tutoring program. The student was being taken out of the class so often for special help that he was losing the continuity of his elementary classroom. The basic skills department lost funding for that student, and staff members were angry that their (quite complicated) removal procedure was ignored. I was actually unaware that there was such a procedure. A conference resulted, which clarified the needs of the basic skills department and also gave our special services team a chance to express our concerns to the department head. In one sense, we were chastised for bypassing procedures; however, we were able to turn a negative event into something positive by using the session for mutual problem solving. Our special services team garnered more respect for the basic skills department and the department was able to appreciate our concerns about excessive pullout programming. We obtained sanction to eliminate pullout for some students as long as we followed the department's procedures.

In New Jersey, this problem also exists in the reverse. Special education students are not supposed to avail themselves of basic skills tutoring because it constitutes "double dipping," which is not permitted when specifically allocated government funds are being used. Yet sometimes, when self-contained students are being prepared for a less restrictive setting, the support of the basic skills class is very important to help the student make the transition from special education classes. Because of the primacy of the individual educational plan (IEP), such flexibility is possible, but only if specified in terms of hours and reasons in the IEP. Consultants who are more systemically oriented may neglect this important microlegalistic step.

In an example affecting the bilingual department, students from Liberia and Jamaica, both English-speaking countries, were being referred for special education when their real problem was a lack of comprehension of *American* English. In a holistic approach to the general problem, the special services team pressed the bilingual department to service these students in ESL (English as a Second Language) classes to help them become used to American-language structures. When the team was able to document specific American-language needs, the bilingual department accepted some of these students, thereby eliminating the need for referral and special education classification.

As part of a consultation project aimed at language stimulation, another problem involved the need for special education tutoring for an entire group of third graders. Regulations prohibited non-classified students from receiving these funded services. One solution was to mix classified and nonclassified students in the special tutor's caseload, as the district was mandated to place students in the least restrictive setting. A setting is defined as less restrictive if classified students are participating with nonclassified students. Another solution was to press the district to develop "open resource rooms" where nonclassified students could benefit from special education services. This required a special designation school by school. If special education students needed the resource room, they could "bump" the nonclassified students. Such bumping only occurred later in the school year, and in the meantime, many non-special education students benefited from the additional services. Of course, pull-*in* programs are preferable to taking children out of their classes. Special education staff working in regular classes can maximize their effect not only by helping the targeted student, but also by coordinating with the regular education teacher to facilitate student learning. Then even more students benefit from the training and modeling that occur. Such pull-in programs usually start at the *system* level (Meyers's Level IV), move to Level III (because they help improve the regular teacher's knowledge and skills, personal growth, and objectivity), and finally go to Level II (where the teacher becomes proficient at gathering objective data, such as assessing growth in students' verbal skills).

In attempting to increase mainstreaming of special education students in a junior high school, our special services team arranged to have some of the students attend regular classes for one or more periods of the day. We obtained a ruling that during those periods, other students could fill the special education slots that had been vacated. If 11 "Neurologically Impaired" students (the maximum in New Jersey) were in such a class, and two went out for one class period each, then another two classified students could avail themselves of that class during those periods, thereby easing the waiting list at the time for special classes. Hence, the consultants, by being innovative and thinking holistically, served more than the two students who were originally mainstreamed.

Another problem of designated funding in some districts is the planning for minor subjects such as art and shop. Their funds are sometimes based on regular class enrollment, not inclusive of the special education enrollment. Because only enough teachers and classrooms are set aside for regular enrollees, attempts to mainstream special education students in these classes are thwarted by legitimate overcrowding. Some union contracts set a maximum number for these classes. Such a problem existed at a junior high in our district. No solution was found, but special services personnel are urged to be aware of such problems when student placement is at issue.

Possible solutions could lie at Meyers's Level IV, where the consultant would intervene with the administrators who plan for class size and number of teachers needed by a school. One problem in our district is that the planning for special education and regular education classes takes place separately, with the two departments rarely communicating. A possible role for the consultant here is to foster communication through meetings with principals and administrators. Intervention could also occur at Levels II and III by working with teachers to devise ways of accommodating the larger load. A Level IV intervention with the union might be required if the contract called for class size limitations.

Some of the above considerations suggest another role expansion for the consultant: that of dealing with state regulatory education agencies. These agencies can often make consultation entry and the general business of educating students more difficult because of regulations that do not consider the in-school realities. For example, such regulations might demand unrealistic paper work, which detracts from the ability to provide more consultation services. Such agencies, as well as legislative bodies, hold hearings or ask for written input from time to time, as they seek to make programs such as special education work better. I urge readers, if they do not already do so, to contribute their thoughts to such agencies. Consultants are on the front line and are aware of problems (and solutions) of which upper-level agencies may be ignorant. Such testimony has had its effects in Pennsylvania and New Jersey, where changes are already taking place to increase preventive efforts and minimize the negative labeling that was previously required in order to provide special education services. The consultant taking a holistic or Level IV systems approach could use schoolwide contacts to mobilize staff opinion and lobby education agencies for changes. This has a negative side as well, because consultants must be careful not to lost their objectivity or step on the toes of sensitive administrators who might prefer to avoid rocking the boat.

One way that a consultant could help students, teachers, and administrators would be to propose alternative, special education in-district programs (and try to obtain the requisite funding) to reduce the numbers of students sent to out-of-district placements. This could save the district a great deal of money and even create teacher and administrator jobs.

In this chapter, we have looked at some nuts-and-bolts problems and solutions so as to alert the consultant to some practical issues that are easy to overlook while designing consultation interventions. We have looked at why it is worthwhile to collect the variety of schedules available in a school. I have emphasized the importance of finding rooms in which to meet, a significant problem in schools where crowding is once again taking place, as special programs and enrollments increase. The differences between consulting at elementary and secondary levels can affect entry, and the consultant who wants to be effective must consider the psychology of the staff at each level. Other issues relating to the location of rooms, departments, and teachers have been explored as they relate to easing consultation entry.

The consultant who desires to be effective tries to cope with the vagaries of school schedules, unexpected meetings and programs, fire drills, arbitrary rules, and designated funding binds. In summary, the creative consultant "works" the system to maximize benefit for the students. Such a consultant sees the possibilities and tries to go beyond the individual student's needs to find a more holistic solution to the problem.

IV

CULMINATION OF EFFECTIVE ENTRY

9

Empowering School Staff: Making Consultation Happen

If consultation work is to have a lasting effect, it should mobilize school staff and resources to carry on the efforts of the consultant. This means creating an environment in which school staff function more effectively by contributing to each other's problem solving. In Meyers's (Parsons & Meyers, 1984) conceptualization of consultation, consultants focus on Level III and IV interventions, because they want to change teachers and the rules and system in which they operate.

In this chapter I discuss the use of school and community resources to aid in consultation. Finding such resources is especially important as the consultant becomes more successful and as greater demands are made for consultation services. The advent of the school resource committee to cope with student problems is explored. The need to make administrators, especially principals, more effective in their work is posited, and that thought is expanded to involve encouraging teachers to provide more leadership and mentoring to make schools more effective.

The practical issue of finding more time to consult is explored, as are issues of role expansion. Special services teams cannot consult creatively unless they are willing to stretch their job, professional definitions, and limitations. I also discuss the need for the consultant to engage constantly in public relations to make the field more accepting and fertile for consultation entry.

UTILIZING RESOURCES

Entry into a school can be eased by the consultant's knowledge of resources. In order to be effective, the consultant helps the school bring together resources from within and without the school to make it run better. Mobilizing resources is also important for the consultant involved with special education, to prevent excessive referrals to the special services teams (Fine, et al., 1979). Once consultants "break the ice" with successful entry, their services may be in great demand and they may have to "handle the flood" (Marks et al., 1987, p. 1) of people asking for their services (Fine et al., 1979).

The first task is to become aware of both in-school and out-of-school resources. In-school resources may include tutoring programs by peers or staff, funded programs such as basic skills (Title I remedial programs), bilingual services, counseling services, senior citizen volunteer programs (Tice, 1987), clubs and activities, screening programs, and so on. Knowing that the school has a Junior Reserve Officer Training Corps (ROTC) or an in-school funded work program can make a big difference when helping staff seek options other than classifying students. In our schools, the basic skills staff are skilled remedial teachers with backgrounds in reading and math. They are knowledgeable in screening for reading and math difficulties, so the child study team's learning consultant or psychologist does not always have to do an evaluation to determine a student's achievement levels.

Although vocational–technical programs provide opportunities for student success when a student is not academically oriented, these teachers' skills may be helpful when consulting with an academic teacher. Vocational–technical teachers often have practical techniques for teaching measurement or reading which could help an academic teacher cope. A printing teacher I knew taught a special education student to center material on a page despite the fact that the student never learned basic measurement skills. The teacher used a large grid, essentially graph-type paper, and taught the student to count the numbers of blocks from right to left or top to bottom to determine the center. Such a grid could be placed under a plain sheet of paper on a table lighted from beneath so that centering could be done on nongrid surfaces.

Knowledge of resources also must include *options* for dealing with problems or difficult students. Options can include administrative transfers, which essentially mean placing a student in another class or school. Grade-level teacher meetings are an in-school option in which teachers are assembled to discuss or meet with students to resolve in-class problems. Some schools permit noncredit auditing of classes (with no test or writing requirements), reduced schedules, partial course credits, part-day job or vocational programs, special interest courses or clubs, and so on.

We once had a very angry teenage student who was befriended by a faculty member who ran a school service club. This student became active in the club and ended up doing a variety of public and civic activities, building self-esteem in the process. The consultant had not set this up (and indeed was unaware of such an option), but it is incumbent upon special services personnel who hope to be more effective to become aware of such opportunities to change behavior. Some changes occur perhaps because of the services a particular school activity provides, but in this case, the special interest of the club adviser was also significant.

In another case, the consultant counseled a depressed, suicidal high school student who had artistic aptitude. The counseling was not succeeding, and she only began to progress when teachers helped her market her excellent artwork and arranged for her to attend a summer art program. Perhaps for the first time in years, she began to believe that people cared, and that maybe she had a future after all.

Community resources should also be tapped (Bardon & Bennett, 1974). Counseling or community mental health agencies might set up a satellite center to help meet the needs of students with behavior or emotional problems. Such programs as the Memphis schools' clinics serve as a model for others (Sleek, 1994). Developing contacts with these agencies for out-of-school referrals can also help the consultant modify behavior.

Industries are increasingly joining with schools to provide curriculum assistance and jobs for students. They could also help with career planning issues, especially with the special education population. The Academy programs in the Philadelphia public schools involve a partnership between industry and schools to serve inner-city high school students. Students are placed in a real-life industrial training situation with state-of-the-art equipment and instructors from the school and industry teaming up to provide the best education. Even in poverty-ridden areas where the dropout rate is very high, such programs have a high completion rate. The consultant called in to examine the high school dropout as an issue must be aware of such possibilities in programming.

Cultural agencies could help with racial pride issues through support and education of ethnic groups. Churches, mosques, and synagogues are often untapped resources, perhaps because public schools are sensitive about church–state separation. Yet these religious organizations are often the only community supports available to certain families. Religious and lay leaders are often willing to help with feeding and housing students and families, providing clothing and also counseling support. The consultant interested in preventive issues needs to tap such resources. Many churches have tutoring programs, services for homeless students, or youth groups to provide after-school activities.

City and district health centers are an important out-of-school resource. They can help the pregnant student receive prenatal and childrearing assistance. They can provide medical diagnostic information which can be helpful in managing students more effectively (e.g., coping with the effects of sickle cell trait or managing prescribed medications). Although these centers focus on indirect service to the student (Level II), the holistic consultant will move from such an individually oriented relationship to utilizing the health service to provide more systemic help to the schools. Such help could involve preventive screening programs to improve staff and student health and perhaps a program to decrease student pregnancies. There is a move to base health clinics in schools (Sleek, 1994), and already 500 exist. President Clinton's 1994 Health Plan also pushed for more school-based health services.

Drug treatment facilities could train staff to recognize substance abuse and might provide educational and therapeutic programs for students. In New Jersey, the county Councils on Alcoholism, together with Department of Education and state substance awareness programs, sponsor Student Assistance Counselors and Core teams in the schools to cope with students with substance abuse problems. Such counselors do preventive group work in school classes, and the Core teams even encourage teachers who are facing addiction problems to go for help. The holistically oriented consultant, when evaluating difficulties apparently residing in the student, will take a more ecological view. In doing so, it may become apparent, for example, that some student problems are really problems of teacher and administrator substance abuse. Good, confidential programs available to staff to help with such problems can make a difference in such areas as effective teaching and efficient administration.

Juvenile shelters could provide staff for preventive programs on coping with runaways. Often the courts or police have their own counseling departments, offering services to law-violating youth and their families. Emergency departments of hospitals have suicide prevention teams to help students in crisis. Often these teams will come to a school or visit a home.

Senior citizen agencies can provide volunteer staff (Courson & Heward, 1989) to help with consultation projects, such as data recording for behavior management, tutoring, conditioning studies, clerical help, and so on. Universities can provide students as teacher aides and tutors. In our community, Princeton University students come to the high school three times a week to provide after-school tutoring. Business schools can provide typists and clerical help. Perhaps such assistance also could come from school vocational/business training programs. Civic organizations such as the Masons, Elks, Rotary Club, and Lions Club sponsor student activities or provide needed financial aid, scholarships, and perhaps even career shadowing opportunities.

THE SCHOOL RESOURCE COMMITTEE

School placement committees, intervention assistance teams, and school resource committees (SRCs) are becoming more widespread as research projects (Project LINK, 1989, in Pennsylvania [Iasello, Miller, Moe, & Richards, 1989; Rosenfield & Shapiro, 1989]; Project R.I.D.E. in Montana [Gabriel, 1989]) or new special education regulations require them. Such teams have been pioneered from New Jersey (Lennox et al., 1986; Lennox et al., 1988; Hamway & Elias, 1988) and Ohio (Zins et al., 1988) to Oregon (Edwards, 1988). SRCs are prereferral intervention teams. They are designed to reduce special education referrals in line with the Regular Education Initiative (1988), which states that schools must realign curriculum and approaches to serve all students better rather than segregating them in special education courses. These teams develop knowledge of the above resources as one of a group of tools to better serve students. Such teams, of course, include my own team's efforts, described in this book, which have reduced special education referrals and classifications. However, our team was a special services team, whereas many of the SRCs come out of efforts across school departmental lines, with active participation of regular education staff. Such teams have also proven effective in reducing special education referrals, promoting satisfaction among teachers and students, and improving student behavior (Sindelar, Griffin, Smith, & Watanabe, 1992).

School resource committees include the principal or designee, special services personnel, regular education teachers both academic and nonacademic (Collins et al., 1988), and special education teachers, as well as remedial educators and the like. Their job is to "own" the referred problems instead of passing them on to special services teams. When regular education school staff own the problem, they do not automatically assume that students who are having problems should be excluded from regular education. They accept the responsibility for proper programming for such students and try to find solutions within the means and resources of the school and staff. They do group problem solving to help their colleagues cope with student problems, instead of routinely making referrals to special education. They brainstorm solutions, follow up on recommendations with checks on the effectiveness of the intervention, and are aware of and utilize the resources mentioned above. They bring out the latent leadership in school staffs, create an important sharing opportunity, and mutually provide support to colleagues. Through these committees, teachers come up with their *own* way of conceptualizing problems (Johnson et al., 1988). This is essential to following through on solutions.

Pugach and Johnson (1989, 1990; Johnson & Pugach, 1991) called their variation on such cooperation between teachers peer collaboration. In their program, teachers worked in pairs, rather than in a committee framework, to develop instructional and behavioral interventions. They accomplished these interventions by following a systematic, highly structured dialogue involving reflective thinking, the results of which are recorded in a special record booklet. This program often leads to a better understanding of the problems in the classroom, which is essential if intervention is to be successful. Discussions are tape-recorded to monitor the accuracy of the structured question asking. The interviewing teacher ("facilitator") guides the interviewee partner ("initiator") into discovering patterns in children's behavior, awareness of the interviewee's own emotional reactions, and exploration of the areas in which the teacher does have clear control. Then the peer team generates interventions and an evaluation plan. The next time the two switch roles, so both receive practice at initiating concerns or facilitating the other's reflective thinking. Such peer teaming easily promotes ownership of problem solving and removes the consultant from the expert and gatekeeper role.

The committee approach involves 2 to 3 years of intensive inservice training of staff in consultation techniques, case management procedures, outcome research, and record maintenance. Project R.I.D.E. uses "effective schools practices" taken from the research literature, a schoolwide assistance team (SWAT Team), which *is* an SRC, and a Tactics Bank and video library identifying 40 classroom problems and 200 proven practices to solve them. Only if all three of these options are utilized and fail is a student referred for special education evaluation.

Project LINK is a cooperative effort in Pennsylvania to "link" the state Department of Education, school districts, intermediate units (administrative units responsible for special services teams), special education, regular education, and the colleges. It is not designed to replace special education classes, but rather to provide better services in the mainstream for the mildly handicapped and "at-risk" student. It involves extensive training in collaborative consultation and curriculum-based assessment, and to make that happen, LINK implements an extensive series of training programs, a case management system, and data-based evaluation. It follows the typical steps of the primary consultation methods in the literature but has the advantage of mobilizing administrative support, freeing the on-the-scene consultant from everyday case management issues while creating a collegial environment in the schools to help teachers problem-solve. Lennox et al. (1988) also tried to administratively free their child study teams from routine reevaluations so that time for consultation could be arranged.

With strong support from university personnel and central office staff, such programs can be most useful for coping with the flood of referrals that good consultants generate (Marks et al., 1988). The consultant's skills are utilized to teach the committee members how to consult with teachers and to help them problem-solve. By training teachers and teams (Meyers's Levels III and IV), a holistic effect occurs, with an expanding number of school staff coping more effectively as problems arise. Moreover, these committees make teachers responsible for helping each other, thereby building confidence in their skills and improving staff morale and cohesiveness. This expands the ownership of school problem solving.

MAKING PRINCIPALS MORE EFFECTIVE

The good consultant is a facilitator. He/she makes things happen by energizing others to become more effective. A key target is the principal. Schools run better when principals do well. The special services team can help principals by freeing them to do the creative and essential tasks of getting into the classroom and working with teachers to improve instruction and behavior management. Maher (1986) taught principals time management techniques to improve their "instructional supervisory behavior." He taught self-management and goal setting. He then measured how much time principals spent observing teachers, providing them with performance feedback, and involving them in improving instruction. He found he could help principals reduce nonsupervisory behaviors, as well as change the balance between other supervisory behaviors (such as hiring, evaluation, and program planning) and direct supportive work with teachers.

Thrust and consideration are two characteristics of effective building administrators that tend to occur in "open" school climates (Halpin, 1967). (See Chapter 2.) Halpin (cited by Sergiovanni & Starratt, 1988) states that "thrust behavior is not . . . close supervision, but . . . the principal's attempt to motivate teachers through the example which he personally sets" (p. 86). A principal showing thrust *models* commitment, effort, and persistence in reaching work goals. Consideration is the concern the principal shows for teachers as human beings.

How can the principal be induced to develop such behaviors if they are not present? The consultant can model such behavior for the principal; can review the research showing how these behaviors are effective in running a better school; or can encourage the *engagement* between teachers, principals, and students, which can be the cause as well as the result of effective thrust and consideration. The consultant can teach or model "strategic leadership" (Adams & Spencer, 1986). This requires that the leader facilitate the opening of cultures to new ways of thinking and being. (See Chapter 4.) The consultant is in a unique position to recognize where the school culture can be opened and who is ready to participate.

TEACHING TEACHERS TO LEAD AND MODEL

The good consultant wants to work him/herself out of a job (i.e., help the school work so effectively that the consultant is not needed). This does not mean that the consultant would literally be without a job, for such success will create quite a demand for the consultant's services. Empowering teachers is one means to this end.

The consultant helps create empowerment through establishing respectful and trusting relationships with staff, refusing to be limited by bureaucratic boundaries in responding to their needs, and creating opportunities for intrastaff collaboration (Christenson & Cleary, 1990). These boundaries include artificial divisions between departments (Smith, 1993). Empowerment occurs when the consultant tries to remove hindrances to effective teacher functioning. Such hindrances include incompetent and uncooperative administrators; heavy workload; lack of materials, resources, and funds; and negative attitudes of the public and parents, among others ("An American Teacher," 1992). One empowers by altering systems or facilitating change in individuals to enhance personal functioning of those individuals (Brown, 1988). Brown asserts that empowerment can occur through *advocacy*, which attempts to change the power relationship between organizations and their clients *or members*. Consultation is the means to do this. When we try to remove hindrances, we may create empowerment, but Brown (1988) cautions that the consultant hoping to advocate better be sure there is a fair chance of success before initiating such steps. He further cautions against grabbing at every cause and issue that comes up.

Consultants can advocate through persuasive writing, by brokering resources, or through communicating with administration to try to correct grievances. When teachers were brought together in an inservice program to solve the lack of substitute teachers (Chapter 4), they became empowered because they advocated for themselves. Helping teachers who are short of materials by working to improve the school's purchase procedure (a Level IV intervention) creates empowerment, as does changing unfair school policies.

The exclusion of developmentally challenged students from the Junior ROTC was a source of great pain for one such student. The consultant worked with the school staff to make ROTC attendance for special education students possible. In the process, the ROTC instructors became empowered as they learned to expand the goals and objectives of ROTC training to more people. For example, one ROTC goal is to improve student citizenship and self-pride. When the consultant reframed these goals to fit the needs of the student concerned, it made sense to the instructor, even though the particular student could not fulfill many of the objectives of the course.

Perhaps teachers are hindered most by uncooperative and bureaucratic administrators. (See Chapters 2 and 3.) The consultant must work to create dialogue between teachers and administrators, constantly seeking opportunities for increased communication. This can be done through talking, persuasive memo writing, volunteering for school committee assignments, helping to facilitate groups, and working to provide programming that will be welcomed by these same administrators and yet will also empower the teachers.

A good way to empower is to create teacher leaders. Leaders are everywhere. In large and small schools, there are always people with good ideas who can inspire others. The consultant's job is to find these people, work with them, and facilitate the adoption of their ideas and methods. The effective schools movement (Bickel, 1990) tries to bring out leadership in teachers. It requires total staff involvement with school improvement, autonomy and flexibility in implementing practices, and teacher-directed classroom management and decision making. This movement, which is bringing about broad agreement on what makes for effective schools, is still in its infancy. This gives the consultant many opportunities to develop staff leadership. The efforts may be focused on a major school change initiative (a Level IV approach) or on individual projects (usually at Levels II and III), a good way to start when the projects do not have the impact to affect the entire school or district.

Our example of basic skills staff developing a workshop for teachers on reading methodology (Chapter 4) is one way to give credit to and encourage skilled people to lead. Encouraging teachers through publicity of their methods in a newsletter is another means to build leadership.

Hostile teachers often make good leaders. They are often angry because they have good ideas and are not being listened to. The special services team member can use his/her position and clinical skills to make these people heard. One teacher hostile to child study teams taught industrial arts. He was angry for a good reason. He felt that the teams ignored vocational issues and evaluation in their individual educational plans. The consultant made a strong effort to tune in to this teacher's needs by writing vocational goals and objectives and developing screening methods for entry into the school's vocational programs. These methods included not only traditional vocational aptitude and interest tests, but also reading samples from the schools vocational texts. This teacher then became receptive to working with the special services team. Later, when he was promoted to an administrative position, he was willing to help the special services team with vocational evaluation of special education students. More important, he was willing to help develop a more comprehensive program of cooperation between special education and the industrial arts department. His leadership and commitment to improving a key program came about because of sensitive cultivation of these skills by the consultants.

Modeling good teaching, or the master teacher concept, can also be encouraged by the consultant. Special services teams can identify good teachers and work with principals to set up inservice programs showcasing the teacher's work. We videotaped exemplary teachers in classroom management settings at an elementary school. We showed the videotapes at one of our workshops, where the same teachers served as a panel of discussants, along with the special services team members, who encouraged participation. The teachers in the audience enjoyed it, as their peers were doing the sharing. They also enjoyed the mistakes these model teachers made, who thereby shared their humanness. Such modeling encourages others to improve, to share, and to discuss teaching.

The consultant can also model. Inviting teachers to attend group counseling (with permission from the group, of course), or doing such counseling in their classroom, provides them with models for communication techniques such as reflection, interpretation, restatement, mirroring, summarizing, and other group methods designed to help students communicate more effectively. The consultant can share leadership with teachers in conducting structured preventive groups in such areas as social skills training, management of aggression, and affective education.

Teacher study groups to review research can also help. For example, teachers who are motivated to improve control in their classrooms can read articles that review the research on student misbehavior (Duke, 1978). Such programs, and those that build skills in peer teaming (Johnson & Pugach, 1991) can accomplish objectives such as increasing teacher control, "with-it-ness" (the ability to be constantly tuned in to what students are doing) (Kounin, 1970), tolerance for students who deviate from the norm, and problem-identification abilities, so that proper interventions can occur. These programs can encourage teachers to teach others. Although the consultant might start off by leading such groups, it is good to encourage rotating leadership as another means of developing leadership skills and a sense of teacher ownership of the group program.

In one school, two teachers started the Learning/Teaching Collaborative (Boles & Truen, 1992). Their goals were to (1) improve education, (2) collaborate with colleges to improve teacher education and lower the teacher–student ratio at the school, (3) eliminate pullout programs and thereby better serve special needs students, and (4) give teachers a means for advancing in their careers (self-actualization motives). They implemented a team teaching approach and got the principal to agree to a restructuring the master class schedule so the teachers could meet for 2 hours a week to plan and participate in a 5-hour Saturday workshop once a month. Such planning time made it possible to revise the curriculum. The addition of new full-time interns lowered the teacher–student ratio so that special needs students could be more readily accommodated. This new ratio gave teachers time to research and write curricula. They also negotiated alternative professional teaching time so they could have time off to do research, mentoring, and teacher training (coupled with a college professor).

A project like this one includes what is called reflective practice. Instead of being "production workers" who expeditiously move students toward graduation while filling them with information, teachers are encouraged to think more deeply about what they do and why they do it (Wellington, 1991; Johnson & Pugach, 1991). To do reflective thinking, teachers need to expand their skill in cognitive reflection (Sparks-Langer & Berstein Colton, 1991). Such skill is developed through self-analysis of video- and audiotapes, by writing postteaching reflective journals, and by action research. Critical reflection includes ethical issues and asks why teachers teach the way they do or why schools require certain methods of teaching. Such thinking challenges competitive grading and some discipline (or behavior control) methods (Sparks-Langer & Berstein Colton, 1991). Teachers write narratives about how they use writing and intentional talk to improve classroom practice and heighten the *awareness of their own professional reasoning.*

Wellington (1991) fosters such reflective thinking through the use of Smyth's (1989) empowerment method, which asks the following:

1. What do I do?
2. What does this mean (in terms of principles or theories)?
3. How did I come to be this way?
4. How might I want to do things differently?

This method, then, requires (1) careful description, (2) informing ourselves, (3) confronting the issues, and (4) reconstructing our practice as teachers. An example might be that the teacher spends 15 minutes of a 45-minute reading class on lecture, 10 minutes on reading a selection from the book, 15 minutes on a worksheet dealing with comprehension issues, and the remaining 5 minutes on setup and cleanup. To answer, "What do I do?" the teacher examines this structure and also the process of how it takes place (content of lecture, the kinds of reading material, and the types of questions asked in the worksheet).

Then the teacher tries to determine what this means. What is the basis in the research for splitting up the time this way? Are there better ways to improve reading levels? Next the teacher asks, "How did I come to be this way?" In a sense, there is a confrontation between the teacher's values and those of the system, between the research and the actual practice. Finally, the practice is reconstructed and changed in line with the new philosophies or goals.

Wellington (1991) views this self-empowerment (which a consultant can certainly encourage) as a kind of defiance of the system akin to "a wildflower growing in the cracks of a concrete and glass city" (p. 5). The teacher, by thinking deeply, is constantly questioning the system. Just as in advocacy, there are risks in attempting empowerment by this method. It is hoped that the consultant has opened the doors of administration sufficiently to allow some of this fresh air to enter.

The consultant also needs to encourage more research by teachers.

Such research can relate directly to consultation outcomes. For example, Sager (1991) encouraged groups of teachers to do research on consultation-related projects. Sager arranged for them to be trained in research methods by university staff and had "critical friends" help them. Such friends could be educators who have research experience, along with administrators and consultants who have *no stake* in the problem being studied. The topic studied was whether writing about math concepts helps to improve math comprehension. The project worked well because of the following:

1. *Volition.* The teachers were working on a topic *they* felt was important.
2. *Availability.* The teachers appreciated the access to these "critical friends," who provided highly qualified free consultation.
3. *"First-class environment."* The training took place in top hotels, and good food reinforced the project's importance.
4. *Public affirmation.* Approval came from colleagues working on the project and those who witnessed it.
5. *Strategic scheduling.* The training took place at times when teachers were least busy.

Empowering others via the "turnkey" concept is being used in the Trenton, New Jersey, schools to teach staff to cope with suicidal behavior: A small number of staff were originally trained by the Community Mental Health Center staff of the University of Medicine and Dentistry of New Jersey and given practice in teaching the workshops; then these "turnkey staff" set up workshops for a wider group, exposing them to communication and listening techniques and diagnostic and referral skills. Teachers who participate in such workshops become leaders themselves and gain new respect from their peers for their knowledge and capabilities.

The turnkey concept can help the overloaded special services team or consultant to manage the "flood" of service demands. Consultants should not try to be everything to everyone. It is better to train others, delegate skills and responsibilities and help the whole system improve.

FINDING TIME TO CONSULT

Many members of special services teams (i.e., inside consultants) have told me that the ideas in this book are sound, but they really have no time to implement them. Johnson et al. (1988) found that special education staff spend little time actually consulting. Although I empathize with the heavy load often carried by special services teams, I have found that careful planning can make consultation quite possible.

One general principle is simply blocking off time. If the consultant has a heavy load of student evaluation assignments, he/she should schedule them only on certain days and never vary. This should leave other days open to doing consultation. In a typical 40-week school year, there are probably at least 35 intact weeks (without holidays, etc.). Spending 2 days per week doing evaluations would net 70 completed cases, sufficient to meet the demands of most heavily burdened urban districts, and certainly adequate for less busy settings.

A second technique is to combine required special education reevaluations with consultation. This can be done through curriculum-based assessment (CBA) (Shapiro, 1987; Shapiro & Derr, 1990; Deno, 1985; Gickling, Shane, & Croskery, 1989) in which samples of classroom work, often from students' own basal readers and math texts, are taken. The student is tested with these samples or "probes" and retested later to check for progress. Probes are done in the easy part of the students' text, in the middle, and at the end, in effect, to tap into independent, instructional, and frustration levels. Spelling probes are developed from the *reading* material, thereby making such learning more relevant, This can often be done in the classroom, with guidance from the teacher. CBA can be spread to other students as the teacher sees student progress and the applicability of CBA to tapping into student progress. The probe data can be used by the teacher to modify curriculum and the teaching approach while meeting the requirements of mandated reevaluations.

Classroom observations, required for reevaluation, are another way to begin a consultation project. These observations, instead of being done for their own sake, using various observation tools (the Instructional Environment Scale [Ysseldyke & Christenson, 1986], Devereux Behavior Rating Scale [Naglieri, Le Buffe, & Pfeiffer, 1992], Weller–Strawser Scales of Adaptive Behavior [Weller & Strawser, 1981], Connors Teacher Rating Scales [Connors, 1990], etc.), are selected after a teacher and consultant have discussed concerns and goals for the child. The observation is adapted to the teacher's concerns and opens the door to further discussions of improving the classroom environment, teaching techniques, or student achievement (see Acheson & Gall, 1980; Ysseldyke & Christenson, 1986; Conoley & Conoley, 1988) for good accounts of specific observation techniques.

When evaluation of students is done, it should always consider the students' adaptive skills; that is, those skills that are meaningful for practical survival. Such behavior also includes the knowledge base the student has, which may be different, especially in urban and rural minority settings, from the characteristics measured by normed tests. For consulting to be effective, student strengths, as well as weaknesses, must be determined, for it is by utilizing these strengths that effective teaching can often be accomplished. The measurement of *adaptive* behavior, as part of evaluating intelligence, is also mandated in many states, including California (where no placement in special education classes can be based on standardized intelligence testing) and New Jersey (where standardized testing is permitted but alternative means of student assessment is encouraged).

Working with teachers and parents is also a means of obtaining such data and can lead to openings to use consultation skills. Effective consulting includes helping teachers see what students are capable of. Why not combine efforts to determine one student's adaptive behavior potential with studies of the whole class's adaptive behavior? One way to do this is to assess the speed with which students master material, or the number of repetitions of word lists needed for mastery. This should be helpful to any teacher, as it creates openings for instructional intervention as teachers get to know students' capabilities. It helps teachers become aware of learning principles such as repetition and feedback. Adaptive behavior in the community could also be chronicled in such areas as ability to use public transportation, read timetables or product labels, or handle banking transactions. The consultant's evaluation time is spent more efficiently when focusing on adaptive issues with individuals and entire classes, because more useful data is being gathered.

Special services team evaluations often end up in files gathering dust. Yet the reports probably convey some important instructional recommendations. Consultants should go over their reports with teachers and open the door to some consultative activity. This is another way of making evaluation time count.

Another way of looking at the consultant's time is to see every moment as an opportunity to do consultation. The staff lunchroom is an ideal place for raw data on consultation intervention. So are the hallways, where the consultant might see an aide struggling to keep order, or the main office, where someone may be complaining about a student who chronically cuts class. Such settings are not only chance opportunities to consult, but often may be settings of *choice*, because the consultant can capitalize on the needs of the moment, when staff are likely to be the most receptive and successful intervention the most visible. The other side of the coin is that the consultant is in the spotlight in such settings and needs to be confident in his/her consulting skills.

A recent lunchroom conversation dealt with a proposed move of all ninth graders from the various junior high schools into our single high school, and the reorganization that would have to take place to accommodate them. With all the complaints and concerns that were being voiced, the special services team member had the opportunity to become a part of the process: to attend the meetings dealing with the change and to get to know the people responsible for making the various decisions. This was a good way to have an impact on the school and to use time effectively.

Lakein (1974) illustrates some effective ideas on time management in his book, *How to Get Control of Your Time and Your Life*. He discusses a number of concepts helpful to the busy consultant, including:

1. Plan time daily. Set priorities.
2. Do the most demanding and difficult tasks first. Do not take the easy way out by doing the often less important things first.
3. Do not be a slave to the telephone. Refuse to answer it except at specific times.

Item 1 is Lakein's key concept. He suggests writing out an agenda of things to do instead of flipping through the usual pile of papers on one's desk. This agenda is based on daily planning time set aside to think about what really needs to get accomplished. For consultants, planning an agenda becomes an assertive action to ensure that consultation will take place. Lakein states that no matter how busy one is, it is worth the investment of 15 minutes to $1/2$ hour to plan how to be most effective. The agenda is the consultant's work plan: I adapted Lakein's ideas into a worksheet that has three columns (see Figure 9.1). The first column lists the tasks to be done; the second column lists the priority value of the task; and the third column is used to

Item	Priority	Action
1. See Carlos for counseling	B3	05-24-95
2. Observe Keisha in reading class	B2	3rd period : 05-22-95
3. Set up consultation conference with Mrs. Perry	A3	Wrote her note : 05-18-95
4. Complete monthly statistics	A2	Done : 05-17-95
5. Evaluate Donna and Consuela	B1	05-21-95
6. See Lashawn - crisis counseling	A1	Asked teacher to send him 1st period : 05-17-95
7. Have secretary copy student permanent records	C1	
8. Clear out "to-be-filed" tray	C2	

FIGURE 9.1. Consultant's work agenda.

write the outcome or actions taken to accomplish the goal. The latter gives the consultant a certain record of accountability.

In the middle column the consultant lists the tasks as A, B, or C priorities. *A* priorities are those that absolutely must be done first. These might include a status report for the boss due today, or a research proposal with a deadline this week. *B* priorities are those that have to be done but do not have the urgency of the A tasks. They might be scheduled reevaluations, team meetings, or class observations. *C* priorities are those that are least important, but that often take up time. They could include opening junk mail, cleaning the coffee pot, listing travel expenses, or filing things that are helpful but not really necessary. If the consultant decides that consultation activities should become A priorities, he/she will write them in the plan as such and will find that the time does exist to do consulting.

The numbers that follow the tasks further clarify the priorities: An A1 task has to be done ahead of A2 and A3. It takes some time to make decisions as to which of these are most important, and the values assigned to each task may vary from day to day. In this list, the consultant has decided that Lashawn's crisis was the most important concern, followed by the monthly report and the consultation conference. The least critical issues, but nonetheless things the consultant would like to get done, were copying records and filing.

Setting priorities is something like the "triage" activities of emergency medical teams. In a crisis, they set aside three areas in a hospital or at an accident or battlesite. Patients are quickly classified as they come in according to the seriousness of their injury, the most serious going to the first area. This way, the emergency personnel's efforts are funneled most efficiently. Consultants also need to focus their efforts so to be sure to attack the most significant problems of the school first. With Lakein's prioritizing method, consultants can remember what needs to be done but can focus on what is most important to them. The agenda ideally should be revised daily, and at a minimum on a weekly basis.

Helping teachers find more time for consultation activities is equally important. The National Education Association's Center for Innovation (1992) surveyed its members to find out how they find time to do all the planning necessary for the restructuring required in the effective schools movement (mentioned earlier in this chapter). Teachers used such methods as the following:

1. *Purchased time.* The district pays teachers for use of their vacation time, or a fund pays for substitutes.
2. *Borrowed time.* Each school day is lengthened by a few minutes

so students can eventually be released for a partial day of teacher planning. In team teaching (see Boles & Truen, 1992), members alternate between teaching and planning.

3. *Common time.* Here the entire day is rescheduled so several teachers will have the same free period. This was done at one of our junior high schools so that we could have grade-level teacher meetings (e.g., all the seventh-grade teachers).

4. *Freed-up time.* Student teachers, parents, community members, volunteers, or administrators take over classes.

5. *Better-used time.* Most of faculty meeting time is devoted to planning instead of announcements or administrative details.

6. *New time.* This is an innovative way of compensating teachers. When teachers use their own time to participate or plan, they receive inservice credit toward continuing education requirements or salary upgrades.

7. *Rescheduled time.* The school calendar is changed to provide for more teacher planning days.

Knowledge of these options can give consultants leverage to help with improving teacher and school effectiveness. It will also help deal with any resistance to setting aside the time necessary for good consultation and planning.

ROLE EXPANSION

Special services personnel have to be open to role expansion if they are to be seen as more than gatekeepers for special education (Ysseldyke, 1984). Consultants must not be trapped by their training and job description, for these can become self-limiting beliefs (Adams & Spencer, 1986). Expanding the consultant's role means lending expertise to school problems that are outside the normal area of practice. Amedore and Knoff (1993) refer to this as "boundary spanning" (p. 343). Such activity often occurs when the consultant's task is especially challenging and "uncertain" (p. 348). Boundary spanning involves using additional people and resources from within or outside the school, with which the consultant typically has not interacted. Even when doing traditional assessment, the consultant can begin to do service delivery in the classroom environment, and expand this by drawing in parents, principals, and others (Piersal, cited in Bergan, 1985). Piersal further states that role expansion can mean doing informal assessments in the classroom or conducting a problem-solving behavioral consultation related to the formal evaluation conducted. Caplan (1970) discusses some of the more accepted roles for a would-be consultant, including:

1. Extending the consultee's "cognitive" field to see that there are systematic ways of dealing with confusing problems.
2. Helping consultees master feelings by legitimizing them and sharing similar feelings the consultant has had.
3. Reducing perceptual distortions (i.e., distortions of what people perceive or expect of, for example, racial or religious groups or even members of other professions).

However, Caplan lists additional roles that represent role *expansion* beyond what many consultants typically do. These represent interventions at more systemic levels (Meyers's Levels III and IV) and include:

1. Improving communication by building trust between competing supervisors or teachers.
2. Improving leadership by being a sounding board for principals or directors and helping leaders to involve staff in real problem solving.
3. Increasing congruence of personal and organizational needs by helping the schools develop policies that take the individual into account.
4. Improving individual and group interpersonal skills.

The holistic, systems-oriented consultant will look for a variety of Level IV means to expand to more flexible roles.

Schmuck (1990) saw the consultant in the following roles:

1. *Action researcher:* Collecting data to help specify and solve problems, encouraging principals to solicit feedback about their leadership styles, and leading staff in goal-setting exercises such as the Delphi method (which includes brainstorming discussions that help set goal priorities) (Schmuck, 1990).
2. *Staff developer:* Changing school norms, structures, and procedures that impede effectiveness, often by organizing training, conducting workshops, coaching administrators in their role, and facilitating the work of teacher committees.
3. *Social architect:* Building cooperation and collaboration, starting "Quality Circles," and improving skill at running meetings.
4. *Political strategist:* Building coalitions with key people to make the school more effective, often becoming an intergroup communi-

cator, mediator, or facilitator; helping the superintendent build more effective public relations by utilizing students and teachers as public relations agents; and working with the superintendent's board or cabinet to help their own team building and meeting improvement.

Consultants can also expand into program evaluation roles (Borich, cited in Bergan, 1985). Borich asserts that good consultants can work with administration to help determine the legitimacy of program goals. Are the goals realistic and will the intervention produce the desired results? Consultants can often uncover mismatches between program intentions and measures of outcome by helping consultees ask the right questions about their intentions (Schein, 1987). Further, they can help determine the appropriateness of program goals to meeting community values and needs so programs will serve the many and not just the few (Borich, cited in Bergan, 1985; Sarason, 1982).

Consultants might feel at this point that they are not sufficiently trained in some of these techniques. Formal training is not necessarily a prerequisite to attempting organizational development (OD) consulting. In a survey of 308 consultants who were doing OD in the schools, Schmuck (1990) found that 50% were inside consultants with little or no formal OD training or linkage to outside experts. In other words, these consultants were taking risks in expanding their traditional roles into Level IV interventions using only the techniques for which their profession trained them. We would need to evaluate to see whether they were really competent in their work. However, I believe that the training of most special services teams is at least a foundation for beginning a holistic approach to their work. It is certainly incumbant upon consultants to obtain the best training they can to improve their skills in working with organizations. I believe such a time investment will be well worth it in terms of job security and satisfaction.

PUBLIC RELATIONS

In order to be effective, special services staff and consultants also need to be attuned to public relations. Yanowitz (1984) and Kelly (1986, 1990) have been writing and speaking for some time now about the importance of public relations. Although they focus on school psychologists, all special services personnel need to be aware of just how visible they are and what kind of professional image they convey.

Image-building activities are similar to role expansion activities because they require consultants to think about their impact beyond the basic services they provide: counseling, testing, or even consulting. Consultants can increase their visibility by being introduced at staff meetings and relating what they do, by serving on school committees, by writing for student and staff newsletters, or by making liaisons with the PTA. Consultants can call parents with good news, provide releases for the local media, make administrators and boards aware of their activities, and let people know who they are by greeting them in hallways and staff lounges. Public relations goals are accomplished when consultants involve key staff in their meetings, join in school events such as picnics, share teacher activities and priorities, and serve as a resource for teachers. One school psychologist offered to be a speaker for the high school's parent–teacher organization (Wedam, 1993). Many parents were surprised at the offer, and some had not even known that there was a psychologist based at the school. Acknowledging the principal's authority and keying work to the principal's needs is a public relations strategy. Simply put, consultants should think of how each activity they do impacts others, and make it have a purposeful result.

SUMMARY

In this chapter I have attempted to pull together the consultant's functions as they affect the system of the school. I have stressed the importance of utilizing resources so that the school becomes more effective in its functioning. This requires efficient allotment of the consultant's time, a flexible view of the consultant's role, and the use of clinical skills to better communicate with administrators, principals, and teachers. Above all, the consultant should strive to be an effective facilitator of school growth and communication.

Throughout this book, I have attempted to convey the difficulties and challenges facing the consultant who desires entry in schools to do consultation. I have shared some of my own experiences in the Trenton, New Jersey, schools, and supplemented it with the work of many other writers. I have used Meyer's framework for finding targets for consultation and have stressed Tom Jackson's views of working to further supervisors' and administrators' goals in order to succeed with the consultant's agenda. I organized the book according to the important people with whom the consultant must deal in order to enter the schools. I have emphasized greatly the role of principals, while also noting the special importance of supervisors, teachers, and support staff; their needs, concerns, and priorities; and how to change them to become more receptive to consultation. I have discussed how critical it is for the consultant to be cognizant of school culture and climate issues. I have noted the importance of parental and community involvement, suggested behavioral and systemic approaches to involvement of parents, and emphasized their importance as a constituency for the consultant.

Barriers, in the form of resistance to consultation, were explored—both external and within the consultant. Effective special services team functioning is critical to the consultation effort, and I have suggested ways of looking at the consultant's team and improving its functioning as well as that of school meetings. Logistical problems that often frustrate consultants, including finding time to consult, were discussed along with ways to overcome these difficulties. School resources must be fully tapped, and the consultant needs to network to promote the image of the consultant and come to know the key people with whom he/she must deal. The importance of the consultant developing good communication skills was stressed.

The consultant must culminate his/her efforts by empowering school staff, whether administrators, teachers, or support personnel. Such activities require role flexibility and expansion on the part of the would-be consultant, and a willingness to be aware of new developments and stretch his/her skills. Above all, one needs patience and the willingness to invest the time to become a part of the school culture, while taking small steps toward a more holistic impact on improving school functioning.

APPENDIX A
Communication Techniques
in Brief

When we talk to people, we want them to listen; conversely, they themselves want to be heard. Consultants and special services personnel require good communication skills if they are to succeed at entry. Accomplishing this is not hard if a few simple techniques are followed. They are easy to learn but take practice if consultants are to come across as sincere (Carkhuff, 1983; Fine et al., 1979; Rogers, 1965). Listening and communication skills have become increasingly important in consultation training programs (see Idol & West, 1987; Horton & Brown, 1990), because of the assumption that they result in successful consultations. However, Horton and Brown (1990) cautioned that most studies of the facilitative characteristics of consultants focused on consultee satisfaction, which does not necessarily mean that the consultation worked. Bergan and Tombari (1976) and Kratochwill and Bergan (1990) are among the few who have used actual problem resolution as the criterion for measuring consultation success.

COMMUNICATION SKILLS IMPORTANT
TO CONSULTANTS

West, Idol, and Cannon (1989) and Knoff, McKenna, and Riser (1991) identified many personal and interactive skills critical for consultant effectiveness in collaborative consultation. Forty-seven consultant skills are included in a Needs Assessment Instrument developed by West, Idol, and Cannon (Figure A.1). Consultants should fill out this questionnaire themselves to determine their need for further training in consultation and communication techniques. This questionnaire includes skills of collaborative problem solving, systems change, equity issues, and values/belief systems, as well as the ability to evaluate consultant effectiveness.

Knoff et al. (1991) developed their consultant skills list by having trainers and practitioners in school psychology rate the characteristics and skills of

Name _____ Position _____

School/Unit _____

Instructions: The skills listed below have been determined by a national panel of experts to be essential for teachers, support staff, and administrators engaging in collaborative consultation for the benefit of handicapped and at-risk students. Please read each skill carefully. Then *rate your need for training* in each skill using the scale listed below. Thank you for taking your valuable time to complete this instrument so that we may better respond to your training needs.

Training Needs Rating Scale

1 = High (1st priority)

2 = Above Average (2nd priority)

3 = Average (3rd priority)

4 = Below Average (4th priority)

5 = None (lowest priority)

CONSULTATION THEORY/MODELS

General and special educators engaging in collaborative consultation will:

_____ 1. Practice reciprocity of roles between consultant and consultee in facilitating the consultation process.

_____ 2. Demonstrate knowledge of various stages/phases of the consultation process.

_____ 3. Assume joint responsibility for identifying each stage of the consultation process and adjusting behavior accordingly.

_____ 4. Match consultation approaches to specific consultation situations, settings, and needs.

RESEARCH ON CONSULTATION THEORY, TRAINING, AND PRACTICE

General and special educators engaging in collaborative consultation will:

_____ 5. Translate relevant consultation research findings into effective school-based consultation practice.

PERSONAL CHARACTERISTICS

General and special educators engaging in collaborative consultation will:

_____ 6. Exhibit ability to be caring, respectful, empathic, congruent, and open in consultation interactions.

_____ 7. Establish and maintain rapport with all persons involved in the consultation process, in both formal and informal interactions.

_____ 8. Identify and implement appropriate responses to the stage of professional development of all persons involved in the consultation process.

_____ 9. Maintain positive self-concept and enthusiastic attitude throughout the consultation process.

_____ 10. Demonstrate willingness to learn from others throughout the consultation process.

_____ 11. Facilitate progress in consultation situations by managing personal stress, maintaining calm in time of crisis, taking risks, and remaining flexible and resilient.

FIGURE A.1. Needs Assessment Instrument. From West, Idol, and Cannon (1989, pp. 299–301). Copyright 1989 by Pro-Ed. Reprinted by permission.

_____ 12. Respect divergent points of view, acknowledging the right to hold different views and to act in accordance with personal convictions.

INTERACTIVE COMMUNICATION

General and special educators engaging in collaborative consultation will:

_____ 13. Communicate clearly and effectively in oral and written form.

_____ 14. Use active on-going listening and responding skills to facilitate the consultation process (e.g., acknowledging, paraphrasing, reflecting, clarifying, elaborating, summarizing).

_____ 15. Determine own and others' willingness (readiness) to enter consultative relationship.

_____ 16. Adjust consultation approach to the learning stage of individuals involved in the consultation process.

_____ 17. Exhibit ability to grasp and validate overt/covert meaning and affect in communications (perceptive).

_____ 18. Interpret nonverbal communications of self and others (e.g., eye contact, body language, personal boundaries in space) in appropriate context.

_____ 19. Interview effectively to elicit information, share information, explore problems, set goals and objectives.

_____ 20. Pursue issues (e.g., problems/situations) with appropriate persistence once they arise in the consultation process.

_____ 21. Give and solicit continuous feedback that is specific, immediate, and objective.

_____ 22. Give credit to others for their ideas and accomplishments.

_____ 23. Manage conflict and confrontation skillfully throughout the consultation process to maintain collaborative relationships.

_____ 24. Manage timing of consultation activities to facilitate mutual decision making at each stage of the consultation process.

_____ 25. Apply the principle of positive reinforcement to one another in the collaborative team situation.

_____ 26. Be willing and feel confident enough to say, "I don't know . . . let's find out."

COLLABORATIVE PROBLEM SOLVING

General and special educators engaging in collaborative consultation will:

_____ 27. Recognize that successful and lasting solutions require commonality of goals and collaboration throughout all phases of the problem-solving process.

_____ 28. Develop a variety of data collection techniques for problem identification and clarification.

_____ 29. Generate viable alternatives through brainstorming techniques characterized by active listening, nonjudgmental responding, and appropriate reframing.

_____ 30. Evaluate intervention alternatives to anticipate possible consequences, narrow and combine choices, and assign priorities.

_____ 31. Integrate solutions into a flexible, feasible, and easily implemented Action Plan relevant to all persons affected by the problem.

_____ 32. Adopt a "pilot" problem-solving attitude, recognizing that adjustments to the Action Plan are to be expected.

_____ 33. Remain available throughout implementation for support, modeling, and/or assistance in modification of the Action Plan.

_____ 34. Redesign, maintain, or discontinue interventions using data-based evaluation.

_____ 35. Use observation, feedback, and interviewing skills to increase objectivity and mutuality throughout the problem-solving process.

FIGURE A.1. (*cont.*)

SYSTEMS CHANGE

General and special educators engaging in collaborative consultation will:

_____ 36. Develop role as a change agent (e.g., implementing strategies for gaining support, overcoming resistance).

_____ 37. Identify benefits and negative effects that could result from change efforts.

EQUITY ISSUES AND VALUES/BELIEF SYSTEMS

General and special educators engaging in collaborative consultation will:

_____ 38. Facilitate equal learning opportunities by showing respect for individual differences in physical appearance, race, sex, handicap, ethnicity, religion, socioeconomic status, or ability.

_____ 39. Advocate for services that accommodate the educational, social, and vocational needs of all students, handicapped and nonhandicapped.

_____ 40. Encourage implementation of laws and regulations designed to provide appropriate education for all handicapped students.

_____ 41. Use principles of least restrictive environment (LRE) in all decisions regarding handicapped students.

_____ 42. Modify myths, beliefs, and attitudes that impede successful social and educational integration of handicapped students into the least restrictive environment.

_____ 43. Recognize, respect, and respond appropriately to the effects of personal values and belief systems of self and others in the consultation process.

EVALUATION OF CONSULTATION EFFECTIVENESS

General and special educators engaging in collaborative consultation will:

_____ 44. Ensure that persons involved in planning and implementing the consultation process are also involved in its evaluation.

_____ 45. Establish criteria for evaluating input, process, and outcome variables affected by the consultation process.

_____ 46. Engage in self-evaluation of strengths and weaknesses to modify personal behaviors influencing the consultation process.

_____ 47. Use continuous evaluative feedback to maintain, revise, or terminate consultation activities.

FIGURE A.1. (*cont.*)

effective consultant behavior and then factor-analyzing the 75 skills into 5 factors based on responses from practitioners. The factors are:

1. *Consultation process skills:* Risk taking (being willing to experiment), promptness of feedback, specification of contract, active role taking for the consultant, pursuit of issues, and ability to confront without attacking.
2. *Expert skills:* Knowledge, questioning skills, good communication skills, good rapport, and conflict resolution.
3. *Personal characteristics:* The ability to practice ethically, problem-solve, and be interpersonally competent, encouraging, and flexible.
4. *Interpersonal skills:* Expressing warmth, encouraging ventilation, being deferent, and maintaining an "I'm OK, you're OK" stance.

5. *Consultant directiveness:* Being confronting, challenging, colorful, and funny.

Knoff also had expert consultants rate the 75 skills; and found that they rated the factors differently from the practitioners. The expert's responses resulted in a Professional Respect factor and excluded the Consultant Directiveness factor.

Parsons and Meyers (1984) consider such directiveness to be critical especially when consultants must deal with resistance on the part of the consultee. Parsons and Meyers specified three forms of confrontation: didactic, experiential, and "calling the game" (after Berne, 1964). Didactic confrontation involves corrective feedback, which is objective, not blaming; an example might be the consultant pointing out an increased loudness of the consultee's voice. Such loudness could reflect resistance, even if the consultee has verbally agreed with the consultant. Experiential confrontation points out conflicts between what the consultee says and does or between different things the consultee said. For example, "You sounded very interested in proceeding with this project, but it seems it has been hard for you to actually get started." "Calling the game" tries to confront any hidden agendas the consultee has respectfully. An example of a game is when the consultee always has an excuse or reason for not carrying out what was agreed to but does not acknowledge any real objections—Berne's (1964) "Yes, But" game. Thus, the consultant might say, "I sense there is a part of you that really is uncomfortable with what we had proposed doing."

In a similar approach to confrontation, Ellis (1962) examines "dysfunctional beliefs of clients." Here, in a Level II intervention (indirect services to the student), one looks at (1) the antecedent behavior (say, a problem behavior of the student), (2) the belief structure or cognitive interpretation of the consultee, and (3) the consequent attitude or feeling the consultee has about the student. A consultee may be angry at a student because she is disrespectful, and the consultee believes that the student must really dislike him/her. The reality may be that the student likes the teacher but needs to test whether the teacher means what he says. Such interpretation or reframing moves the consultation to Level III, because the consultant is seeking change in the teacher's cognitions.

Bergan and Tombari (1975) developed a model for examining communication that takes place between consultant and consultee. They examined message content, processes, and control. The content includes the topics covered in the consultation, such as student background and specific behaviors. The processes focus on the kinds of consultant verbalizations specified by West, Idol, and Cannon (1989) as interactive skills. These include clarification, interpretation, and summarization. The message control category specifies verbalizations from the consultant that either provide information *to* or elicit information or action *from* the consultee; that is, the consultant attempts to *control* the verbalization that comes from the consultee so that the consultee learns to specify important data.

The importance of process skills and interpersonal skills had been recognized by Tombari and Bergan (1978) who stressed the examination of *language* skills in consultation problem resolution. Although their analysis focuses on how to speak to a teacher, the approach applies equally to principals, supervisors, and others with whom the consultant is likely to consult. They stress the value of focusing on "behavior" rather than on "problems" as a means of increasing optimism in consultees.

Putting together the recommendations of the above studies, it would appear that the consultant needs:

1. *Personal characteristics:* A caring, approach and the ability to facilitate progress in consulting by being calm, taking risks, and being open-minded and flexible. The consultant must be trustworthy and well-adjusted, and maintain confidentiality.

2. *Process skills:* The ability to identify clear and common goals and be aware of relationship issues such as power, dependency, and role clarification. The consultant must develop a variety of data collection techniques and use observation, feedback, and interviewing skills to increase objectivity and mutuality while engaging in collaborative problem solving.

3. To be a *change agent:* Using directiveness and confrontation, if necessary, to impact on the consultee and the system, to promote equal learning opportunities, and to modify myths about the integration of handicapped students into the least restrictive, inclusive environment. To be an effective change agent, consultants must use humor and aggression and must be colorful, challenging, and self-disclosing (Knoff et al., 1991). It may also involve control skills.

4. *Control skills:* Being sure that what is said is eliciting the most effective responses from the consultee (Bergan & Tombari, 1975). Here the consultant operationalizes the process of communication by studying both process and content. This means looking at the message source, its content, and the message control elicitors or emitters. When interviewing, the consultant uses elicitors to try to get the consultee to specify exact behavior descriptions. For example, "How often does Ronald get out of his seat?" Then the consultant uses behavior-*setting* specification elicitors to bring out the antecedent, consequent, and sequential conditions connected with the student's behavior.

ASSESSING COMMUNICATION IN THE CONSULTING SESSION

While it is a good idea for consultants to try to rate their skills on Figure A.1, they must also assess how they handle face-to-face consultation sessions. A good checklist for examining what has been discussed with a principal (or teacher) at a meeting is presented in Figure A.2. Rosenfield suggests tape-re-cording the initial consultation interview and then rating and tallying each of the consultant's responses to the consultee according to the categories on the checklist. The tallies are then converted as percentages of all responses and examined to see if too many questions were asked, if the consultant switched to different areas without pinning down all the information needed in one area, or if paraphrasing, clarifying, and perception checking were used (see below for more on these terms). Rosenfield then recommends that consultants set goals for improving their use of communication skills.

Conoley and Conoley (1982) present another good checklist of personal process (communication) skills (see Figure A.3). This checklist may also be useful in analyzing a tape recording or videotape of the consultant's behavior in a consultation session. The list is helpful because it provides a scale on which consultants, their supervisors, or their team members can rate their skills. It does not limit the consultant to an either/or category, and as such it becomes a more formative means of evaluating skills. After practice in consulting, the form could be filled out again to ascertain progress (e.g., in improving empathy or the ability to confront).

When doing a behavioral consultation, consultants might use Kratochwill and Bergan's (1990) Problem Identification Interview Data Sheet (Figure A.4) to clarify which objectives they pursued and what the consultee's responses were. Here consultants check off whether they have information on all the items required for a successful behavioral consultation. These include, among others, the opening salutation and the response to it, as well as specification of the target behaviors with examples and priorities, sequential conditions, and summarization and validation of what has been said. The Occurrence column is used to note whether each objective occurred, and the Response column to note what the consultee's response was to that objective. These decisions can be made by objective observers, or the consultant can tape a session and judge for him/herself. The reliability of such judgments, if made by more than one person, can be recorded at the top of the form in the space allocated. The "general statement" noted on the data sheet is an introduction to the consultation, such as, "Mr. Snyder, you referred Tamika because of her difficulty concentrating on her school work?" After this general statement, the consultant tries to have the behavior of concern clearly spelled out with examples, and to clarify the consultee's priorities (i.e., under behavior specification and behavior setting). To continue our example, Tamika's concentration problem would need to be specified in observable terms: "She looks out the window when I lecture." Antecedents in this case would be those events that preceded her looking out the window, and sequential conditions those that accompany this behavior (such as who Tamika is sitting with, what time of day it is, etc.). Consequent conditions are identified by asking what happened after the behavior of concern. Behavior strength refers to how

	Tally	Total	%
1. Requesting Clarification			
2. Paraphrasing			
3. Perception Checking			
4. Active Listening			
5. Asking Focused, Relevant Questions			
6. Offering Information			
7. Examining Child's Work			
8. Asking Irrelevant Questions			
9. Other			

FIGURE A.2. Record sheet for monitoring consultation sessions. From Rosenfield (1987, p. 231). Copyright 1987 by Lawrence Erlbaum Associates. Reprinted by permission.

1.	7	6	5	4	3	2	1
	Expresses affection (can say positive, supportive statements to another)						Does not express affection
2.	7	6	5	4	3	2	1
	Accepting (nonjudgmental, nonevaluative)						Not accepting
3.	7	6	5	4	3	2	1
	Flexible (varies behaviors according to the situation)						Inflexible
4.	7	6	5	4	3	2	1
	Pursues issues (once issues arise, stays with them)						Drops issues
5.	7	6	5	4	3	2	1
	Empathic (is sensitive to other's emotional states)						Nonempathic
6.	7	6	5	4	3	2	1
	Congruent (consistency between) feelings and behaviors)						Noncongruent
7.	7	6	5	4	3	2	1
	Able to confront (ability to confront group and individuals with salient issues)						Unable to confront
8.	7	6	5	4	3	2	1
	Self-disclosing (open, clearly states own feelings)						Closed

FIGURE A.3. Personal process skills form for consultants. From Conoley and Conoley (1982, pp. 16–18). Copyright 1982 by Pergamon Press. Reprinted by permission.

9.	7	6	5	4	3	2	1

Able to live with stress (able to function in the presence of intense emotions) — Unable to live with stress

10.	7	6	5	4	3	2	1

Perceptive (level of understanding/insight and ability to communicate these) — Nonperceptive

11.	7	6	5	4	3	2	1

Listens well (ability to grasp meaning and affect in communication) — Listens poorly

12.	7	6	5	4	3	2	1

Sums up well (ability to summarize and facilitate movement) — Sums up poorly

13.	7	6	5	4	3	2	1

Resilient (ability to hang in and bounce back) — Nonresilient

14.	7	6	5	4	3	2	1

Caring (concern for others) — Not caring

15.	7	6	5	4	3	2	1

Views self positively (quality or self-image) — Views self negatively

16.	7	6	5	4	3	2	1

In touch with own aggressive feelings (ability to admit and check punitive, purely self-enhancing responses) — Not in touch with aggressive feelings

FIGURE A.3. (*cont.*)

17.	7	6	5	4	3	2	1
	Expresses aggression effectively (confronts others without personal attacks)						Too punitive or too mild
18.	7	6	5	4	3	2	1
	Able to anticpate (intervenes with awareness of possible consequences)						Unable to anticipate
19.	7	6	5	4	3	2	1
	Distancing (appropriate personal involvement that facilitates communication)						Distancing ineffective (too close or too far away)
20.	7	6	5	4	3	2	1
	Takes risks (willing to experiment with new behavior)						Does not take risks

FIGURE A.3. (*cont.*)

often behavior occurs and how long-lasting it is. When the consultee summarizes and validates, he/she feeds back what the consultee seemed to have said about the behavior and its consequences or its strength, for example, "You stated that Tamika looks out the window 90% of the time when you are giving a class lecture, and when you call it to her attention, she turns around briefly, but then watches what the other children are doing."

Goals for behavior change are defined and assets identified (what the student is good at). Existing procedures are identified (how much time is given to class lecture?), and again this information is summarized and checked for accuracy with the consultee. Next a directional statement must be made to explain which data it is important to record on this student's behavior and why, and it is decided how the data will be collected. Agreement on this is summarized and validated and a date set to begin recording, and one for the next consultation. This 20-item data sheet gives a good sense of how effectively the consultant elicited important information about the behavior and the setting in which it took place.

Consultants should use these checklists to test how they have handled a given consultation. They can use the items to increase their awareness of how they interact with teachers as well as with principals, supervisors, and other key people in the entry process.

Date: _____ Observer: _____

Client: _____ Reliability: _____

Consultee: _____ Observer: _____

Consultant: _____ Session #: _____

Interview objective	Occurrence	Response
1. Opening salutation		
2. General statement		
3. Behavior specification		
a. Specify examples		
b. Specify priorities		
4. Behavior setting		
a. Specify examples		
b. Specify priorities		
5. Identify antecedents		
6. Identify sequential conditions		
7. Identify consequences		
8. Summarize and validate		
9. Behavior strength		
10. Summarize and validate		
11. Tentative definition of goal		
12. Assets question		
13. Question about existing procedures		
14. Summarize and validate		
15. Directional statement about data recording		
16. Data collection procedures		
17. Summarize and validate		
18. Date to begin data collection		
19. Establish date of next appointment		
20. Closing salutation		

FIGURE A.4. Problem Identification Interview Data Sheet. From Kratochwill and Bergan (1990, pp. 107–108). Copyright 1990 by Plenum Press. Reprinted by permission.

A CLOSER LOOK AT LISTENING
AND RESPONDING SKILLS

Let us look more carefully at how consultants can examine and practice the kinds of listening and responding skills that are important. Rosenfield (1987) cites Bergan's recommendation to practice recognizing the categories of communication and then to rehearse them, using, for example, Carkhuff's categories of attending, responding, personalizing, initiating, and action (Carkhuff et al., 1983). Learning each category will help consultants improve in the areas Knoff et al. (1991) listed as important (i.e., process skills, developing a sense of calm, self-disclosing, and eliciting skills).

Are you aware of *attending* well to what the consultee says? Attending refers to the physical context and your body language; observing the consultee's levels of energy, feelings, and intellect, and listening nonjudgmentally. Attending requires making eye contact, positioning oneself facing the consultee, and being sure to listen "actively" (Rosenfield, 1987) in order to have accurate data when one responds. Attending also means recognizing the signs that a consultee does or does not want to talk at that moment.

Once consultants show that they are tuned in, they need to respond. In *responding* one should be tuned to both content and feelings. Responding also requires being supportive, sensitive to the emotional state of the consultee, congruent (meaning that one's feelings and behavior must be consistent), and self-disclosing (Conoley & Conoley, 1982), as well as asking relevant questions (Rosenfield, 1987; Kratochwill & Bergan, 1990).

The consultant must then also *personalize* the discussion by connecting the topic to the consultee's life and how his/her goals relate to the situation.

West, Idol, and Cannon (1989) broke down. Responding and Personalizing into the following elements:

1. Acknowledging
2. Paraphrasing
3. Reflecting
4. Clarifying
5. Elaborating
6. Summarizing

Acknowledging is the simplest level of Responding, and like Carkhuff's attending might include a simple nodding of the head or a "yes." Paraphrasing, reflecting, clarifying, and elaborating are all included in Carkhuff's responding. Paraphrasing is putting the other person's words in the consultants own as a test of whether the consultant heard correctly. Reflecting techniques are like paraphrasing, and they essentially mirror what has been said so that the person knows he/she has been heard. The quality of this reflection is such that the person does not regret that the information was shared. That is, it is a nonjudgmental comment that shows what the consultant heard. An example of reflecting when consulting with a principal might be:

PRINCIPAL: The Curriculum Coordinator sent another directive about our achievement scores being below the state standards.
CONSULTANT: It seems like the administration is really pressuring you to raise student test scores.

This is a nonjudgmental statement that is put out for verification. If it is correct, it may stimulate more sharing. If incorrect, it leaves things open for the principal to clarify. In any case, it is better than jumping in with one's own opinion:

CONSULTANT: I think this emphasis on test scores is ridiculous!

This may be a true expression of the consultant's feeling (and even reflect the current thinking in the field) but it ignores what the person is saying and may close off communication.

The next level of Reflecting is to look for the feeling *behind* the words. This is riskier, because the consultant is guessing what a person feels. Hence the communication must be put in more tentative terms, and again should not be judgmental:

CONSULTANT: It sounds like you are really angry about the pressure from the administration, with this new emphasis on test scores.

Such a response tells the consultee that the consultant is trying to tune into his/her feelings and gives the person the opportunity to expand on the feeling, or clarify:

PRINCIPAL: No, I'm not really angry, just frustrated that they expect higher scores, when we're dealing with kids who have so many societal handicaps. I wish we had more control over what goes on at home.

This opens the door to exploring how the school could intervene in problems at home and leaves the principal receptive to discussions with the consultant about what to do next. The consultant's response was open enough that the principal could indicate concern about control of environmental factors rather than solely express anger.

Effective communication also involves clarifying. Here one goes beyond mirroring and attempts to obtain a clearer picture:

CONSULTANT: Do you really mean that the school could fail its evaluation if even one classroom does not pass the California Achievement Test?

Clarifying statements can help communication too. The tactic here is to "play dumb." It is not necessarily game playing, nor is it insincere, for we often make the mistake of saying we understand, just to be polite, when we really do not know exactly what a person is getting at. Rosenfield (1987) noted that consultants often do not ask for clarification and assume that they understand what is being said about the consultation issue. For example:

PRINCIPAL: I'm really annoyed that the administration keeps sending memos about our school's achievement test scores.
CONSULTANT: Yeah, I know what you mean.

How often have we said something like that? A common response in social conversation, the result of a statement like this could be the end of the conversation or deterioration into a mutual griping session. A better statement might be: "I don't quite follow you," or "Can you explain that further?" or "How do you mean?" Such open-ended requests for clarification would elicit further details about the consultee's priorities, worries, or agendas, which opens up more possibilities for consultation entry.

Elaborating is carrying the consultee's remarks further. If the principal clarifies that the school missed passing the evaluation because of the failure of five classrooms on the test, the consultant might respond as follows:

CONSULTANT: So it seems that you might need to find a way to increase the test scores of at least five classes.

Such elaboration must also be tested by reality, by constantly looking to the consultee for verification. Elaboration brings us back to Carkhuff's categories, because it is similar to his Initiating step, in which the consultant begins to operationalize, or create workable objectives for, the personal concerns just identified. In Initiating as well as Elaborating, the consultant attempts to show the consultee that there are practical means for pursuing his/her concerns (see Kratochwill & Bergan, 1990). Elaborating falls short of actually making recommendations, because it carries forward the consultant's *interpretations* of what the consultee appears to be thinking and feeling.

Finally, verbal communication requires Summarizing. This is another technique to show that the consultant has heard what was said. Here the consultant summarizes the main points of a discussion out loud and again asks for verification:

CONSULTANT: So I gather we may need to do more work with the students' familes to help improve test scores.

In the case of a consultation with a teacher over a students' behavior:

CONSULTANT: So it appears our main concerns are with Randall's out-of seat behavior and with the need to move him from writing complete sentences to paragraphs of four to five sentences. How does that fit with your own impressions of our session?

Carkhuff would then proceed to the *action* step, in which the operational aspects of the Initiating step become translated to specifics that consultant and consultee would do:

CONSULTANT: We have agreed that you will observe the frequency of his out-of-seat behavior, and I will gather data using the observation scale we reviewed on how you sequence your writing lesson so we can set goals for our next consultation.

Note the resemblance of these communication techniques to the first five steps in the consultation process (see Chapter 1): entry, problem definition, problem analysis, goal setting, and implementation. In order for consultation to proceed well, the skills of communicating need to be in place as a *kind* of foundation for basic entry and the detailed stages that follow. These communication categories, necessary to good interpersonal relations, probably should be mastered prior to learning the critical steps in problem identification and problem analysis. The careful search for definable objectives, operational definitions of problems, goal specification, and spelling out performance objectives that occur in the consultation process (Kratochwill & Bergan, 1990) require tuning in to what consultees are saying and helping them express more precisely what they mean: hence the need to acknowledge, paraphrase, reflect, clarify, and summarize the content and the feelings of the consultee.

Such communication skills are also necessary in the later consultation stage of evaluation. In behavioral consultation there is more of a focus on objective data than on feelings, which are emphasized more in collaborative consultation. A look at a transcript of an evaluation interview that followed a behavioral consultation (Kratochwill & Bergan, 1990, pp. 170–174) reveals a great respect for the consultee and his/her ability to come up with options. In the transcript, the teacher, trying to get a nonverbal child to verbalize more, tells the consultant that the method he/she tried did not work. The consultant acknowledges, paraphrases, and reflects, but quickly gets to the stage of initiating action by clarifying information about what the student likes and later summarizing what will be done:

CONSULTANT: Okay, how did it go?

CONSULTEE: Well, it's not working.

CONSULTANT: It's not working! [acknowledges; reflects]

CONSULTANT: (after some further discussion) How often did he talk? [clarifies]

CONSULTEE: Just about three times. That's about it.

CONSULTANT: Three times in a whole week? [paraphrases; clarifies]

CONSULTEE: Yes. (*then later*)

CONSULTANT: What we did was indirect. I think we need to try something that's more powerful. Is there anything around the school that Walter likes? [summarizes past attempt; initiates new proposal; clarifies] (*still later*)

CONSULTEE: I could do something like give him a piece of candy or something like that when he talks.

CONSULTANT: You could do that? You could give him candy? [paraphrase and reflection] (*later*)

CONSULTEE: When he points to something.

CONSULTANT: Right. When he points, you could say, "Walter, if you say 'paint,' I'll give you the paint." [acknowledging; elaborating]

Some of the clarifying is of what the *consultant*, not the consultee, is saying. This is also important in good communication because the consultant has a responsibility for being sure his/her message comes across clearly.

A different emphasis is noted in a collaborative approach used by Rosenfield (1987) during instructional consultation. The problem shown below is "Danny's" academic difficulties, which the consultant more appropriately refers to as academic "behaviors," a focus similar to behavioral consultation.

TEACHER: Well, Danny is a great break dancer. He's not too bad in math. Sentence writing he's not too good in, neither is his grammar. Reading is his worst problem. His comprehension and phonic skills are very poor . . .

CONSULTANT: Tell me more about his reading problem. [Here the consultant focuses on one key area by acknowledging and asking for clarification] (*later*)

TEACHER: I call his name and he pays no attention. He stares out the window.

CONSULTANT: Sometimes it's difficult to reach a child and we try all sorts of things. [reflection of feeling; elaborating by showing understanding that the teacher has tried many alternatives]

TEACHER: I just don't know what's going on with him. Some days he can do most of the work, and other days he's just out of it. His family life doesn't help.

CONSULTANT: It's a trying situation. [reflection] You mentioned earlier that he has problems in writing. Can you tell me something about his writing? [attending; clarifying]

Here the consultant shows awareness of the pain the teacher is experiencing, shows she has been listening by recalling a problem mentioned at the start of the interview (writing), and then seeks further clarification of that problem.

I used Carkhuff's approach with a supervisor of our special services team. The steps were as follows: Using *Attending* skills, I perceived my new supervisor's concerns about the need to pursue the suicide prevention program, regarding which the district's training had become inactive. I *Responded* (using reflection, clarifying, and summarizing) to the feelings of anxiety about the possible consequences of not continuing such a program and to the content of her statements about the need for details on how to proceed. *Personalizing* took the form of defining her perceptions of what was needed, as well as sharing my own concerns, which paralleled hers. Relating the matter to specific cases we had worked on also helped to personalize the discussion. We determined what she wanted to do, which was to emphasize the program at the high school level. The *Initiating* step was to operationalize the program: agree on what steps should be taken (inside or outside people to do the training, who to do it, whom to train, what materials would be used, and what would follow the training). We then agreed on *Actions* to be taken by each of us: who would call the trainers, who would approve the trainer fees, who would convene a meeting of staff at the high school, who would contact the principal and special education director, and so on.

If consultants undertake these actions, the assumption is that they want to be helpers (Carkhuff, 1983) and are willing to listen, negotiate, and pitch in their own efforts when gathering the fruits of listening to and exploring the supervisor's needs. This is also consistent with Tom Jackson's (1977) guerrilla tactics, designed to help the supervisor become more effective.

For these techniques to work, there must be a "genuineness": on the part of the consultant (Gutkin & Curtis, 1990). Rigid, unspontaneous verbalizations will be ineffective if not said with warmth and true empathy. Nonverbal behavior of the consultant can also give away insincerity. Consultants should look at their body language, including how they physically set boundaries in the space between them and their consultees.

In summary, there must be an attempt to get into the other person's shoes and feel what they are feeling, not in a *diagnostic* sense but rather in a supportive, caring manner. Even clinically trained consultants often come across as too diagnostic:

CONSULTANT: You are having angry feelings.

This statement tone puts the consultee in the patient chair and comes across as cold and analytical instead of indicating that the consultant is a warm person who cares about what the consultee is saying. Such reflective statements should be assiduously avoided. A better response might be:

CONSULTANT: *(said caringly)* I can sense how steamed up you feel about this issue. It must really get to you.

Another type of communication comes under *assertive* behavior. This is used to explain a point of view in a way that is most likely to be accepted. The "I" statement followed by a feeling is a good way to express this.

CONSULTANT: I enjoy doing inservice projects with school staff. [or] I like to analyze data, and would find it an interesting challenge to review the discipline records to see if we could identify any patterns.

Assertive behavior, which Curtis and Meyers (1985) sometimes refer to as confrontation, is also needed when the consultant's goals are being compromised too much, or if there is excessive resistance to steps that have already been agreed to (Caplan, 1970; Parsons & Meyers, 1984). Consultants can often be assertive while sounding puzzled:

CONSULTANT: It seems we had agreed to set up regular meetings with the second-grade teachers, but nothing yet has happened in that regard.

Here the consultant is confronting a principal with the lack of action on a preagreed step but is not being hostile or blaming.
The "I" approach can also be used here:

CONSULTANT: I am feeling really frustrated that there has been no progress on setting up the inservice we talked about.

Confrontation can involve an interpretation of what is really happening to block the consultative efforts. With the above principal, the consultant might state:

CONSULTANT: I wonder if you are having some doubts about this inservice idea, since nothing yet has happened to get it started.

When confronting a teacher who has not followed through on an agreed change to a more assertive stance, because she seems to be uncomfortable about being an authority with her new students, Curtis and Meyers (1985) suggest that the consultant might say:

CONSULTANT: Let's spend a few minutes thinking about what you just said. Do you think it implies that one important issue might have to do with your own ambivalence about being an authority figure to the students?

Dealing with principals in this objective, reflective capacity may be difficult, especially for the inside consultant who is also struggling with the principal's authority demands. It may also be hard to speak this way with teachers the consultant knows well, because social conversations do not typically involve such confrontation.

Consultants should role play, listen to tapes, and check themselves out by obtaining feedback from consultees. Continual use of these communication skills will help any consultant become more effective.

APPENDIX B
The School Climate Survey

Instrument Description: This survey, developed by the Pennsylvania Department of Education, was designed to gather information on a wide range of school climate topics. Respondents could include teachers, administrators, students (above grade seven), and parents. The survey includes: Part A, General Climate Factors; Part B, Program Determinants; Part C, Process Determinants; and Part D, Material Determinants. Within each of the parts, groups of three items represent a sub-area. For example, the first three items in Part A are concerned with the area of respect. The next three items are concerned with trust. It should take about 20 minutes to complete the survey in most cases. Responses to each item are 1, Almost Never; 2, Occasionally; 3, Frequently; and 4, Almost Always. Respondents indicate "What should be" and "What is" for the school for each item.

Why Use This Instrument: Administering this instrument is a reasonable way of gathering data on a wide range of school climate topics. The four major sub-areas were noted above. A total of 24 sub-areas are included in the instrument. Since respondents are to identify what is and what should be, the survey identifies areas that need improvement. In scoring, the "What is" scores should be contrasted to the "What should be" in order to establish a discrepancy. Establishing a discrepancy may help to motivate some people to narrow that gap between what is and what should be.

Using and Scoring the Instrument: Each respondent completes the survey independently, responding to the items with a 1 to 4 value on a Likert scale. Each item has two scores the "What is" and "What should be" responses. Mean scores are calculated for the school based on the groups responding and for the total group of respondents. Scores should be analyzed for the 24 sub-areas found on the survey and for the four major parts of the survey. Special emphasis should be placed on the analysis of scores illustrating the discrepancy between what is and what should be. This could be done by graphing the scores using a what is line and a what should be line, or through a series of histograms. Norms are not available for this survey.

Suggested Activities: Graphs could be provided to the school staff indicating the results outlined in the previous sections. Staff members could analyze the re-sults to identify those areas where the "What is" scores were at an unsatisfactory level. Also, the discrepancy scores could be reviewed to locate areas that need improvement. A list of those items that can be improved based on the resources available should be established. From that list priorities could be established and the school staff could work to improve in those areas over 1 to 2 years.

From Pennsylvania Department of Education (1988, pp. 31–39).

SCHOOL CLIMATE SURVEY

Attached is a list of statements about your school. Tell us if you agree or disagree that the statements describe your school. Be honest. Do not tell us your name.

1. Please answer these questions first:

   I am a: (check one)

		Sex (circle one)	
____ Student	Grade ____	Female Male	

		Sex (circle one)	Years Taught (circle one)
____ Teacher	Grade(s) Taught ____	Female Male	1-5 6-10 11-15 16-20 over 20

	My child is in	Sex (circle one)	
____ Parent	Grade ____	Female Male	

   ____ School Staff Member (e.g., secretary, custodian, librarian or nurse)

   ____ Administrator in this school

   ____ Administrator from Central Office

2. Fill out the rest of the pages this way:

EXAMPLE

Read each sentence. To the right are two columns marked "What Is" and "What Should Be." Circle the number in each column that tells how you feel about your school. For the example, "Teachers treat students with respect," a "3" circled in the first column means this is frequently true <u>right now</u> at your school. The circled "4" in the second column means teachers <u>should almost always</u> respect students.	What Is: 1--Almost Never 2--Occasionally 3--Frequently 4--Almost Always	What Should Be: 1--Almost Never 2--Occasionally 3--Frequently 4--Almost Always
1. Teachers treat students with respect.	1 2 3 4	1 2 3 4

Thank you for your help. We will use your answers to make your school a better place for everyone.

Part A
General Climate Factors

	What Is: 1--Almost Never 2--Occasionally 3--Frequently 4--Almost Always	What Should Be: 1--Almost Never 2--Occasionally 3--Frequently 4--Almost Always
1. Teachers treat students with respect.	1 2 3 4	1 2 3 4
2. Teachers from one subject area or grade level respect those from other subject areas.	1 2 3 4	1 2 3 4
3. Teachers in this school are proud to be teachers.	1 2 3 4	1 2 3 4
4. Students feel that teachers are "on their side."	1 2 3 4	1 2 3 4
5. Students can count on teachers to listen to their side of the story and to be fair.	1 2 3 4	1 2 3 4
6. Teachers trust students to use good judgment.	1 2 3 4	1 2 3 4
7. Students are enthusiastic about learning.	1 2 3 4	1 2 3 4
8. Attendance is good; students stay away only for urgent and good reasons.	1 2 3 4	1 2 3 4
9. Teachers like working in this school.	1 2 3 4	1 2 3 4
10. I feel that my ideas are listened to and used in this school.	1 2 3 4	1 2 3 4
11. Important decisions are made in this school with representation from students, faculty and administration.	1 2 3 4	1 2 3 4
12. When all is said and done, I feel that I count in this school.	1 2 3 4	1 2 3 4
13. Teachers in this school seek better ways of teaching and learning.	1 2 3 4	1 2 3 4
14. Students feel that the school program is relevant to their future needs.	1 2 3 4	1 2 3 4

15. The school supports parent involvement.
    Opportunities are provided for parents to
    be involved in learning activities and in
    examining new ideas.   1 2 3 4   1 2 3 4

16. Students would rather attend
    this school than transfer to another.   1 2 3 4   1 2 3 4

17. There is a "we" spirit in this school.   1 2 3 4   1 2 3 4

18. New students and faculty members
    are made to feel welcome and part
    of the group.   1 2 3 4   1 2 3 4

19. When a problem comes up, this
    school has procedures for working
    on it.   1 2 3 4   1 2 3 4

20. When a student comes along who
    has special problems, this school works
    out a plan that helps that student.   1 2 3 4   1 2 3 4

21. New programs are adapted to the
    particular needs of this community
    and this school.   1 2 3 4   1 2 3 4

22. There is someone in this school that
    I can talk to about problems.   1 2 3 4   1 2 3 4

23. The principal really cares about students.   1 2 3 4   1 2 3 4

24. I think people in this school care
    about me as a person; are concerned
    about more than just how well I
    perform my role at school (as
    student, teacher, parent, etc.).   1 2 3 4   1 2 3 4

Part B
Program Determinants

	What Is: 1--Almost Never 2--Occasionally 3--Frequently 4--Almost Always	What Should Be: 1--Almost Never 2--Occasionally 3--Frequently 4--Almost Always
1. Students help to decide learning objectives.	1 2 3 4	1 2 3 4
2. Teachers are actively learning.	1 2 3 4	1 2 3 4
3. This school's program stimulates creative thought and expression.	1 2 3 4	1 2 3 4
4. Each student's special abilities (intellectual, artistic, social, or manual) are challenged.	1 2 3 4	1 2 3 4
5. All students are not held to the same standards.	1 2 3 4	1 2 3 4
6. Teachers know students as individuals.	1 2 3 4	1 2 3 4
7. Individual and small-group settings, as well as classroom-sized groups, are used in this school.	1 2 3 4	1 2 3 4
8. Teachers use a wide range of teaching materials and media.	1 2 3 4	1 2 3 4
9. Teachers and administrators attend inservice education programs to support their own growth.	1 2 3 4	1 2 3 4
10. Students are given alternative ways of meeting curriculum requirements.	1 2 3 4	1 2 3 4
11. Teachers are known to modify their lesson plans on the basis of student needs.	1 2 3 4	1 2 3 4
12. Extracurricular activities appeal to students.	1 2 3 4	1 2 3 4
13. The school's program encourages students to develop self-discipline and initiative.	1 2 3 4	1 2 3 4
14. The administration is supportive of teachers.	1 2 3 4	1 2 3 4

15. Faculty and staff want to help every
    student learn.   1 2 3 4   1 2 3 4

16. Teachers and their students together
    work out rules governing behavior in
    the classroom.   1 2 3 4   1 2 3 4

17. Discipline (punishment) when given
    is fair and related to violations of
    agreed-upon rules.   1 2 3 4   1 2 3 4

18. Most students and staff members
    obey the school's rules.   1 2 3 4   1 2 3 4

19. Students know the criteria used to
    evaluate their progress.   1 2 3 4   1 2 3 4

20. Teachers are rewarded for
    exceptionally good teaching.   1 2 3 4   1 2 3 4

21. Most students get positive feedback
    from faculty and staff.   1 2 3 4   1 2 3 4

Part C
Process Determinants

	What Is:	What Should Be:
	1--Almost Never 2--Occasionally 3--Frequently 4--Almost Always	1--Almost Never 2--Occasionally 3--Frequently 4--Almost Always

1. People in this school do a good job of examining alternative solutions before deciding to try one.   1 2 3 4   1 2 3 4

2. Ideas from various community groups are sought in problem-solving efforts.   1 2 3 4   1 2 3 4

3. People in this school solve problems; they don't just talk about them.   1 2 3 4   1 2 3 4

4. Community involvement is sought in developing the school's goals.   1 2 3 4   1 2 3 4

5. The goals of this school are used to provide direction for programs.   1 2 3 4   1 2 3 4

6. The goals of this school are reviewed and updated.   1 2 3 4   1 2 3 4

7. There are procedures open to me for going to a higher authority if a decision has been made that seems unfair.   1 2 3 4   1 2 3 4

8. This school believes there may be several alternative solutions to most problems.   1 2 3 4   1 2 3 4

9. When we have conflicts in this school, the result is constructive, not destructive.   1 2 3 4   1 2 3 4

10. I feel the teachers are friendly and easy to talk to.   1 2 3 4   1 2 3 4

11. The principal talks with us frankly and openly.   1 2 3 4   1 2 3 4

12. Teachers are available to students who want help.   1 2 3 4   1 2 3 4

13. Parents help to decide about new school programs.   1 2 3 4   1 2 3 4

14. I have influence on the decisions within the school which directly affect me.   1 2 3 4   1 2 3 4

15. The student government makes important decisions.   1 2 3 4   1 2 3 4

16. Teacher evaluation provides useful information for improving teacher performance.   1 2 3 4   1 2 3 4

17. Teachers or students can arrange to deviate from the prescribed program of the school.   1 2 3 4   1 2 3 4

18. Teachers are held accountable in this school for providing learning opportunities for each of their classes.   1 2 3 4   1 2 3 4

19. The teachers in this school know how to teach as well as what to teach.   1 2 3 4   1 2 3 4

20. Inservice education programs available to teachers help them keep up-to-date on the best teaching strategies.   1 2 3 4   1 2 3 4

21. The school encourages students to help other students with their learning activities.   1 2 3 4   1 2 3 4

22. In this school we "look ahead;" we don't spend all our time responding to daily problems.   1 2 3 4   1 2 3 4

23. Information is collected and used to help make decisions at this school. Priorities for this school are set by several groups, such as teachers, parents and community leaders.   1 2 3 4   1 2 3 4

Part D
Material Determinants

	What Is: 1--Almost Never 2--Occasionally 3--Frequently 4--Almost Always	What Should Be: 1--Almost Never 2--Occasionally 3--Frequently 4--Almost Always
1. There is sufficient staff in this school to meet the needs of its students.	1 2 3 4	1 2 3 4
2. The instructional materials are adequate for our school program.	1 2 3 4	1 2 3 4
3. Current teacher salaries in this community give fair recognition of the level of professional service rendered by teachers to the community.	1 2 3 4	1 2 3 4
4. Teachers and students are able to get the instructional materials they need at the time they are needed.	1 2 3 4	1 2 3 4
5. Teachers recommend and make judgments about priorities for resources needed in their program.	1 2 3 4	1 2 3 4
6. The support system of this school fosters creative and effective teaching/learning.	1 2 3 4	1 2 3 4
7. The building is kept clean and in good repair.	1 2 3 4	1 2 3 4
8. This school building has the space and physical arrangements needed to conduct the kinds of programs we have.	1 2 3 4	1 2 3 4
9. Students and staff are proud of their school plant and help to keep it attractive.	1 2 3 4	1 2 3 4

References

Acheson, K., & Gall, M. D. (1980). *Techniques in the clinical supervision of teachers*. New York: Longman.

Adams, J. D., & Spencer, S. (1986). Consulting with the strategic leadership perspective. *Consultation: An International Journal, 5*, 149–159.

Aden, J. J. (1991, March). Mobilizing kindergarten parents. *NASP Communique*, p. 24.

Ailington, R. L., & Johnston, P. (1989). Coordination, collaboration and consistency: The redesign of compensatory special education interventions. In R. E. Slavin, N. Maden, & N. Karweit (Eds.), *Preventing school failure: Effective programs for students at risk* (pp. 320–354). Boston: Allyn & Bacon.

Albee, G. W. (1983, Fall). Psychopathology, prevention and the just society. *Journal of Primary Prevention, 4*(1), 5–40.

Albee, G. W. (1984). Prologue: A model for classifying prevention programs. In J. M. Joffe, G. W. Albee, & L. D. Kelly (Eds.), *Readings in primary prevention of psychopathology*. Hanover, NH: University Press of New England.

Alpert, J. L. (1984). School consultation. In J. E. Ysseldyke (Ed.), *School psychology: The state of the art*. Minneapolis, MN: National School Psychology Inservice Training Network.

Alpert, J. L., & Meyers, J. (1983). *Training in consultation*. Springfield, IL: C. C. Thomas.

Alpert, J. L., & Yammer, M. D. (1983). Research in school consultation: A content analysis of selected journals. *Professional Psychology, 14*, 604–612.

Amedore, G. H., & Knoff, H. M. (1993). Boundary spanning activities and the multidisciplinary team process: Characteristics affecting school psychological consultation. *Journal of Educational and Psychological Consultation, 4*(4), 343–356.

An American teacher—A profile. (1992, September). *NEA Today*, pp. 12–13.

Amidon, E. J., & Flanders, N. A. (1971). *The role of the teacher in the classroom: A manual for understanding and improving teacher classroom behavior.* St. Paul, MN: Association for Productive Teaching.

Armor, D., Conry-Oseguera, P., Cox, M., King, N., McDonnel, L., Pascal, A., Pauly, E., & Zellman, G. (1976). *Analysis of the school preferred reading program in selected Los Angeles minority schools* (Report No. R2007–LAUSD). Santa Monica, CA: Rand Corp.

Ashton, P. T., & Webb, R. B. (1986). *Making a difference: Teachers' sense of efficacy and student achievement.* New York: Longman.

Axford, S. (1986). A developmental–ecological approach to conceptualizing social systems [Abstract]. *National Association of School Psychologists Convention Proceedings* (pp. 1, 2). Hollywood, FL: National Association of School Psychologists.

Bardon, J. (1979). Educational development as school psychology. *Professional Psychology, 10,* 224–233.

Bardon, J. (1985). On the verge of a breakthrough. *Counseling Psychologist, 13*(3), 355–362.

Bardon, J., & Bennett, V. C. (1974). *School psychology.* Englewood Cliffs, NJ: Prentice-Hall.

Batsche, G. (1991, December). Schools and families: Forging effective partnerships. *NASP Communique, 20*(4), 2.

Bergan, J. R. (1977). *Behavioral consultation.* Columbus, OH: Charles Merrill.

Bergan, J. R. (1985). *School psychology in contemporary society.* Columbus, OH: Charles Merrill.

Bergan, J. R., & Kratochwill, T. R. (1990). *Behavioral consultation in applied settings.* New York: Plenum Press.

Bergan, J. R., & Tombari, M. L. (1975). The analysis of verbal interactions occurring during consultation. *Journal of School Psychology, 13,* 209–226.

Bergan, J. R., & Tombari, M. L. (1976). Consultant skill and efficiency and the implementation of outcomes of consultation. *Journal of School Psychology, 14,* 3–14.

Berne, E. (1964). *Games people play: The psychology of human relationships.* New York: Grove Press.

Bickel, W. E. (1990). The effective school literature: Implications for research and practice. In T. B. Gutkin & C. R. Reynolds (Eds.), *The handbook of school psychology* (2nd ed., pp. 847–867). New York: Wiley.

Blake, R., & Mouton, J. (1964). *The managerial grid.* Houston, TX: Gulf.

Blum, R. E., Butler, J. A., & Olson, N. L. (1987, September). Leadership for excellence: Research-based training for principals. *Educational Leadership, 45,* 25–29.

Boice, R. (1989). Psychologists as faculty developers. *Professional Psychology, 20*(2), 97–104.

Boles, K., & Truen, V. (1992, February). How teachers make restructuring happen. *Educational Leadership, 49*(5), 53–57.

Borders, L. D., & Drury, S. M. (1992). Comprehensive school counseling programs: A review for policymakers and practitioners. *Journal of Counseling and Development, 70*(4), 487–498.

Bowser, P. B. (1994, March). Special education procedures: When the school psychologist and the special education director disagree. *NASP Communique, 22*(6), 18.

Bronfenbrenner, U. (1979). *The ecology of human development.* Cambridge, MA: Harvard University Press.

Broughton, S. F., & Hester, J. R. (1993). Effects of administrative and community support on teacher acceptance of classroom interventions. *Journal of Educational and Psychological Consultation, 4*(2), 169–177.

Brown, D. (1985). The preservice training and supervision of consultants. *Counseling Psychologist, 13*(3), 410–425.

Brown, D. (1988). Empowerment through advocacy. In D. J. Kirpius & D. Brown (Eds.), *Handbook of consultation: An intervention for advocacy and outreach* (pp. 5–17). Alexandria, VA: Association for Counselor Education and Supervision.

Bunn, T. (1987). Sociological perspective on special education: I. *Educational Psychology in Practice, 2*(4), 5–9.

Calliari, C. L. (1992, September). The mentor's role: Linking novices to resources. *NJEA Review, 10,* 26–28.

Canning, C. (1991). What teachers say about reflection. *Educational Leadership, 48*(16), 18–21.

Canter, L. (1989). *Assertive discipline.* Santa Monica, CA: Lee Canter.

Caplan, G. (1970). *The theory and practice of mental health consultation.* New York: Basic Books.

Carbo, M. (1987a, February). Reading styles research: What works isn't always phonics. *Phi Delta Kappan, 68,* 431–435.

Carbo, M. (1987b, November). Deprogramming reading failure: Giving unequal learners an equal chance. *Phi Delta Kappan, 68,* 197–201.

Carkhuff, R. R., with Pierce, R. M., & Cannon, J. R. (1983). *The art of helping.* Amherst, MA: Human Resource Development Press.

Casanova, U. (1989). Research and practice: We can integrate them. *NEA Today, 7*(6), 44–49.

Casey, A. (1992, March). Site-based management: An opportunity for school psychology. *NASP Communique, 20*(6), 22.

Christenson, S. L., & Cleary, M. (1990). Consultation and the parent–educator partnership: A perspective. *Journal of Educational and Psychological Consultation, 1*(3), 219–241.

Clayton, C. (1988, March). [*Untitled address to the Eighth Annual Conference on the Future of Psychology in the Schools*], Philadelphia, PA.

Cobb, C. (1992, February). Paradigm shift and the focus on outcomes. *NASP Communique, 20*(5), 3–5.

Coch, L., & French, J. R. R. (1948). Overcoming resistance to change. *Human Relations, 1,* 512–532.

Collins, F., Brash, E., Watkin, A., Venhorst, R., & Connolly, M. (1988, December). *Plan to revise special education in New Jersey.* Workshop presented at the winter meeting of the New Jersey Association of School Psychologists, Clark, NJ.

Commission on the Prevention of Mental—Emotional Disabilities. (1987, Summer). Childhood; adolescence. *Journal of Primary Prevention, 7*(4), 209–214.

Connors, K. (1990). *Connors' Teacher Rating Scales.* North Towanda, NY: Multi-Health Systems.

Conoley, J. C., & Conoley, C. W. (1982). *School consultation: A guide to practice and training.* New York, NY: Pergamon Press.

Conoley, J. C., & Conoley, C. W. (1988, November). Useful theories in school-based consultation. *RASE: Remedial and Special Education, 9*(6), 14–20.

Coplin, J. W., & Houts, A. C. (1991). Father involvement in parent training for oppositional child behavior: Progress or stagnation. *Child and Family Behavior Therapy, 13*(2), 29–51.

Corso, M., & Murphy, J. (1988, December). *Chemistry of child study teams.* Paper presented at the winter meeting of the New Jersey Association of School Psychologists, Clark, NJ.

Corwin, R. (1965). Professional persons in public organizations. *Educational Administration Quarterly, 1*(3), 7–12.

Courson, F. H., & Heward, W. L. (1989, May). Using senior citizen volunteers in the special education classroom. *Academic Therapy, 24,* 525–532.

Cowen, E. L., & Hightower, A. D. (1990). The primary mental health project: Alternative approaches in school-based preventive intervention. In T. B. Gutkin & C. R. Reynolds (Eds.), *The handbook of school psychology* (pp. 775–795). New York: Wiley.

Curtis, M. J., & Meyers, J. (1985). Best practices in school-based consultation: Guidelines for effective practice. In A. Thomas & G. Grimes (Eds.), *Best practices in school psychology* (pp. 79–94). Washington, DC: National Association of School Psychologists.

Davis, J. M., & Sandoval, J. (1991). A pragmatic framework for systems-oriented consultation. *Journal of Educational and Psychological Consultation, 2*(3), 201–216.

DeForest, P. A., & Hughes, J. N. (1992). Effect of teacher involvement and teacher self-efficacy on ratings of consultant effectiveness and interaction acceptability. *Journal of Educational and Psychological Consultation, 3*(4), 301–316.

Deno, S. (1985). Curriculum-based measurement: The emerging alternative. *Exceptional Children, 52,* 219–232.

Dowling, E., & Osborne, E. (1985). *The family and the school: A joint systems approach to problems with children.* London: Routledge & Kegan Paul.

Duane, E. A., Bridgeland, W. M., & Stern, M. E. (1986). The leadership of principals: Coping with turbulence. *Education, 107,* 212–220.

Duke, D. L. (1978). The etiology of student misbehavior and the depersonalization of blame. *Review of Educational Research, 48,* 415–437.

Dyke, N., & Dettmer, P. (1989). Collaborative consultation: A promising tool for serving gifted students with learning disabilities. *Journal of Reading, Writing and Learning Disabilities International, 5*(3), 253–264.

D'Zurilla, T. J., & Goldfried, M. R. (1971). Problem solving and behavior modification. *Journal of Abnormal and Social Psychology, 78,* 107–126.

Edwards, J. (1988, November). *Consultation: A mode to enhance school social work practice.* Paper presented at the annual conference of the National Association of Social Workers, Philadelphia, PA.

Eitel-Brown, S., Lamberth, J., & Hyman, I. (1984). Time utilization of school psychologists in Trenton. *Psychology in the Schools, 12*(3), 325–328.

Elliott, S. N. (1988). Acceptability of behavioral treatments in educational settings. In J. C. Witt, S. N. Elliott, & F. M. Gresham (Eds.), *Handbook of behavior therapy in education*, (pp. 121–150): New York: Plenum Press.

Elliott, S. N. (1992, May). Authentic assessment: A critical part of educational reform in the '90's. *NASP Communique, 20*(7), 12–14.

Elliott, S. N., Witt, J. C., Galvin, G., & Peterson, R. (1984). Acceptability of positive and reductive intervention: Factors that influence teacher decisions. *Journal of School Psychology, 22*, 353–360.

Ellis, A. (1962). *Reason and emotion in psychotherapy*. New York: Lyle Stuart.

Ellis, J., & Osowski, J. V. (Eds.). (1990, November). *A plan to revise special education in New Jersey: An overview of pilot project outcomes*. Trenton, NJ: New Jersey Department of Education.

Ellison, G. C., & Burke, J. P. (1987). Strategy for selecting organizational development interventions for schools. *Professional School Psychology, 18*(4), 385–390.

Erchul, W. P. (1987). A relational communication analysis of control in school consultation. *Professional School Psychology, 2*, 113–124.

Erchul, W. P. (1991, March). An interview with Gerald Caplan. *NASP Communique, 20*(6), 18–19.

Erchul, W. P., & Chewning, T. G. (1990). Behavioral consultation from a request-centered relational communication perspective. *School Psychology Quarterly, 5*(1) 1–20.

Erion, J. (1992, June). Parent tutoring, reading instruction and curriculum-based measurement. *NASP Communique, 20*, 15–16.

Facherty, A. C., & Turner, C. D. (1988). Changing at the top? An attempt by educational psychologists to influence special education policy within an educational authority. *Educational Psychology in Practice, 4*(2), 99–104.

Fierson, R. (1987). A model for assessing team meetings. *Clearing House, 8*, 60.

Fine, M., Grantham, V. L., & Wright, J. G. (1979). Personal variables that facilitate or impede consultation. *Psychology in the Schools, 16*(4), 533–539.

Fish, M. C., & Jain, S. (1988). Using systems theory in school assessment and intervention: A structural model for school psychologists. *Professional School Psychology, 3*, 291–300.

Flanagan, D., & King, T. (1980, June). *Parent consultation model*. Paper presented at the annual convention of the Pennsylvania Psychological Association, Lancaster, PA.

Foreman, J. B. (Ed.). (1969). *American gem dictionary*. London: Collins.

Freiberg, P. (1991, January). The guru of prevention calls for social change. *APA Monitor*, 28–29.

French, J. R., & Raven, B. (1959). The bases of social power. In D.

Cartwright (Ed.), *Studies in social power* (pp. 150–167). Ann Arbor, MI: Institute for Social Research.

Friend, M., & Bauwens, J. (1988). Managing resistance: An essential consulting skill for learning disabilities teachers. *Journal of Learning Disabilities, 21*(9), 556–561.

Friend, M., & Cook, L. (1992). The ethics of collaboration, *Journal of Educational and Psychological Consultation, 3*(2), 181–184.

Gabriel, S. (1989). Project RIDE (Responding to Individual Differences in Education) [Abstract]. In A. Cantor & P. Dawson (Eds.), *Directory of alternative service delivery models* (p. 43). Washington, DC: National Association of School Psychologists.

Gagne, R. M. (1977). *The conditions of learning* (3rd ed.). New York: Holt, Rinehart & Winston.

Gallesich, J. H. (1973). Organizational factors influencing consultation in schools. *Journal of School Psychology, 11*(1), 57–65.

Gallesich, J. H. (1982). *The profession and practice of consultation.* New York: Jossey-Bass.

Gallesich, J. H. (1985). Meta-theory of consultation. *Journal of Counseling Psychology, 13*(3), 336–354.

Gallesich, J. H., & Derby, N. J. (1976). *Consultant Assessment Form.* Unpublished evaluation form, University of Texas at Austin, Department of Educational Psychology.

Gersch, I. S., & Rawkins, P. (1987). A teacher support group in school. *Educational and Child Psychology, 4*(3–4), 74–81.

Getting the job done: The pluses and minuses [Profile]. (1992, September). *NEA Today,* p. 13.

Giammatteo, M., & Giammatteo, D. (1981). *Forces on leadership.* Reston, VA: National Association of Secondary School Principals.

Gickling, E. E., Shane, R. L., & Croskery, K. M. (1989). Developing mathematics skills in low achieving high school students through curriculum-based assessment. *School Psychology Review, 18*(3), 344–355.

Gold, R. F., & Hollander, S. K. (1992). The status of consultant teacher services in special education on Long Island, NY: 1989–1990. *Journal of Educational and Psychological Consultation, 3*(1), 25–38.

Gottfredson, G. D. *Effective school battery.* Odessa, FL: Psychological Assessment Resources.

Gottfredson, G. D., & Hollifield, J. H. (1988, March). How to diagnose school climate. *National Association of Secondary School Principals Bulletin, 72,* 63–70.

Graden, J. L. (1989). Redefining "pre-referral intervention": as intervention assistance: Collaboration between general and special education. *Exceptional Children, 56*(3), 227–231.

Graden, J. L., Zins, J. E., & Curtis, M. J. (Eds.). (1988). *Alternative educational delivery systems: Enhancing instructional options for all students.* Washington, DC: National Association of School Psychologists.

Gresham, F. M. (1991). Conceptualizing behavior disorders in terms of resistance to intervention. *School Psychology Review, 20*(1), 23–36.

Gresham, F. M., & Noell, G. H. (1992). Documenting the effectiveness of consultation outcomes. In J. E. Zins, T. R. Kratochwill, & S. N. Elliott (Eds.), *The handbook of consultation services for children* (pp. 249–273). San Francisco: Jossey-Bass.

Grimes, J. (1981, Spring). Shaping the future of school psychology. *School Psychology Review, 10,* 206–232.

Grubb, R. (1981, Spring). Shaping the future of school psychology: A reaction. *School Psychology Review, 10,* 243–259.

Gutkin, T. B., & Bossard, M. D. (1984). The impact of consultant, consultee and organizational variables on teacher attitudes toward consultation services. *Journal of School Psychology, 22,* 251–258.

Gutkin, T. B., & Curtis, M. J. (1982). School-based consultation: Theory and techniques-Intervention in the schools. In C. R. Reynolds & T. B. Gutkin (Eds.), *The handbook of school psychology* (pp. 796–828). New York: Wiley.

Gutkin, T. B., & Curtis, M. J. (1990). School-based consultation: Theory, techniques and research. In T. B. Gutkin & C. R. Reynolds (Eds.), *The handbook of school psychology* (2nd ed., pp. 577–613). New York: Wiley.

Gutkin, T. B., & Reynolds, C. R. (Eds.). (1990). *The handbook of school psychology* (2nd ed.). New York: Wiley.

Gutkin, T. B., & Tieger, A. G. (1979). Funding patterns for exceptional children: Current approaches and suggested alternatives. *Professional Psychology, 10*(5), 670–680.

Haight, S. L. (1984). Special education teacher consultant: Idealism vs. realism. *Exceptional Children, 50*(6), 507–515.

Hallahan, D. P., Kauffman, J. M., Wills Lloyd, J., & McKinney, J. D. (Eds.). (1988, January). Questions about the regular education initiative. *Journal of Learning Disabilities, 21*(1), 3–52.

Halpin, A. W. (1967). *Theory and research in administration.* New York: Macmillan.

Halpin, A. W., & Croft, D. B. (1963). *Organizational climate of schools.* Chicago: University of Chicago Midwest Administration Center.

Hamway, T., & Elias, S. M. (1988, March). *School-based decision-making: The role of the psychologist in intervention assistance teams.* Paper presented to the eighth annual conference on the Future of Psychology in the Schools, Philadelphia, PA.

Harris, A. M., & Cancelli, A. A. (1991). Teachers as volunteer consultees; Enthusiastic, willing or resistant participants? *Journal of Educational and Psychological Consultation, 2*(3), 217–238.

Harvey, V. S. (1989, December). System program evaluations: Feasible and effective. *NASP Communique, 18,* p. 25.

Henderson, A. (1990, December). Beyond the bake sale: Basic principles of partnership between families and schools. *NASP Communique, 19*(4), 24.

Heron, T. E., & Kimball, W. H. (1988). Gaining perspectives with the educational consultation research base: Ecological considerations and further recommendations. *RASE: Remedial and Special Education, 9*(6), 21–28.

Hodges, W. (1980, Spring). An agenda for school psychologists. *School Psychology Review, 10*(2), 290–297.

Holland, J. L. (1966). *Psychology of vocational choice.* Waltham, MA: Blaisdell.

Horton, G. E., & Brown, D. (1990). The importance of interpersonal skills in consultee-centered consultation: A review. *Journal of Counseling and Development, 68,* 423–426.

Hoy, W. K., & Clover, S. (1986). Elementary school climate: A revision of the OCDQ. *Educational Administration Quarterly, 22*(1), 101.

Hoy, W. K., & Miskel, C. G. (1987). *Educational administration: Theory, research and practice.* New York: Random House.

Huebner, E. S. (1992a). Leadership skills for school psychologists: Improving parental involvement in multi-disciplinary team interactions. In S. L. Christenson & J. C. Conoley (Eds.), *Home-School collaboration: Enhancing children's academic and social competence* (pp. 409–422). Washington, DC: National Association of School Psychologists.

Huebner, E. S. (1992b). Burnout among school psychologists: An exploratory investigation into its nature, extent and correlates. *School Psychology Quarterly, 7*(2), 129–136.

Huebner, E. S. (1993). Psychologists in secondary schools in the 1990's: Current functions, training and job satisfaction. *School Psychology Quarterly, 8*(1), 50–56.

Huebner, E. S., & Gould, K. (1991). Multidisciplinary teams revisited: Current perceptions of school psychologists regarding team functioning. *School Psychology Review, 20*(3), 428–434.

Huebner, E. S., & Hahn, B. M. (1990). Best practices in coordinating multi-disciplinary teams. In A. Thomas & J. Grimes (Eds.), *Best practices in school psychology—II* (pp. 235–246). Washington, DC: National Association of School Psychologists.

Huefner, D. S. (1988). The consulting teacher model: Risks and opportunities. *Exceptional Children, 54*(5), 403–414.

Hyman, I. (1974, September). *An overview of problems in consultation.* Paper presented at the annual convention of the American Psychological Association, New Orleans, LA.

Hyman, I., & Dougherty, K. (1988, March). *School climate assessment.* Paper presented at the eighth annual conference on the Future of Psychology in the Schools, Philadelphia, PA.

Iannone, R. (1987). The inner voices of principals. *Education, 107*(3), 326–332.

Iasello, J., Miller, A., Moe, E., & Richards, D. (1989). *Project LINK.* Reading, PA: Berks County Intermediate Unit, Tech and Media Center, Special Education Services.

Idol, L. (1983). *Special educators consultation handbook.* Austin, TX: Pro-Ed.

Idol, L. (1988). A rationale and guidelines for establishing special education consultation programs. *RASE: Remedial and Special Education, 9*(6), 48–58.

Idol, L., Paolucci-Whitcomb, P., & Nevin, A. (1986). *Collaborative consultation.* Austin, TX: Pro-Ed.

Idol, L., & West, J. F. (1987). Consultation in special education: Part II. Training and practice. *Journal of Learning Disabilities, 20*(8), 474–497.

Insel, P. M., & Moos, R. H. (1974). *The work environment scale.* Palo Alto, CA: Consulting Psychologists Press.

Jackson, J., H. (1993, Spring). Practice in urban schools and the overlooked opportunity. *School Psychologist, 47*, 1, 5, 16.

Jackson, T. (1977, October). *Guerrilla tactics in the job market.* Seminar, Fort Washington, PA.

Johnson, L. J., & Pugach, M. C. (1991). Accommodating the needs of students with mild learning and behavior problems through peer collaboration. *Exceptional Children, 57*, 454–461.

Johnson, L. J., Pugach, M. C., & Hammitte, D. J. (1988). Barriers to effective special education consultation. *Remedial and Special Education, 9*(6), 41–47.

Johnston, J. C., & Zemitzsch, A. (1988). Family power: An intervention beyond the classroom. *Behavioral Disorders, 14*(1), 69–79.

Johnston, P., Ailington, R. L., & Afflerbach, P. (1985). The congruence of classroom and remedial reading instruction. *Elementary School Journal, 85*(4), 465–478.

Kelly, C. (1986). Effective public relations at the building level [Summary]. *NASP Convention Proceedings,* pp. 63–64.

Kelly, C. (1990). Best practices in building-level public relations. In A. Thomas & J. Grimes (Eds.), *Best practices in school psychology—II* (pp. 171–182). Washington, DC: National Association of School Psychologists.

Keys, C. (1983). Graduate training in organizational consultation. In J. Alpert & J. Meyers (Eds.), *Training in consultation* (pp. 123–141). Springfield, IL: C. C. Thomas.

Kirpius, D. J. (1985). Consultation interventions: Successes, failures and proposals. *Counseling Psychologist, 13*(3), 368–389.

Knight, M. F., Meyers, H. W., Paolucci-Whitcomb, P., Hasaszi, S., & Nevin, A. (1981). A 4-year evaluation of consulting teacher service. *Behavior Disorders, 6*(2), 92–100.

Knoff, H. M. (1984). The practice of multi-modal consultation: An integrating approach for consultation service delivery. *Psychology in the Schools, 21*, 83–91.

Knoff, H. M., McKenna, A. F., & Riser, K. (1991). Toward a consultant effectiveness scale: Investigating the characteristics of effective consultants. *School Psychology Review, 20*(1), 81–96.

Kounin, J. (1970). *Discipline and group management in classrooms.* New York: Holt, Rinehart & Winston.

Kramer, J. (1990). Training parents as behavior change agents: Successes, failures and suggestions for school psychologists. In T. B. Gutkin and C. R. Reynolds (Eds.), *The handbook of school psychology* (pp. 683–702). New York: Wiley.

Kratochwill, T. R. (1978). *Single subjects research: Strategies for evaluating change.* New York: Academic Press.

Kratochwill, T. R. (1985). Selection of target behaviors in behavioral consultation. *Behavioral Assessment, 7,* 49–61.

Kratochwill, T. R., & Bergan, J. R. (1978). Behavioral consultation model. *Professional Psychology, 9,* 71–82.

Kratochwill, T. R., & Bergan, J. R. (1990). *Behavioral consultation in applied settings.* New York: Plenum Press.

Kratochwill, T. R., & Van Someren, K. R. (1985). Barriers to treatment success in behavioral consultation: Current limitations and future directions. *Journal of School Psychology, 23,* 225–239.

Kune, N. (n.d.). Integration: Being realistic isn't realistic. *Canadian Journal for Exceptional Children, 1*(1), 4–8.

LaCayo, N., Sherwood G., & Morris, J. (1981). Daily activities of school psychologists: A national survey. *Psychology in the Schools, 18,* 184–190.

Lakein, A. (1974). *How to get control of your time and your life.* New York: McKay.

Lambert, N. (1981, Spring). School psychology training for the decades ahead. *School Psychology Review, 10*(2), 194–205.

Lazarus, A. A. (1981). *The practice of multi-modal therapy: Systemic, comprehensive and effective psychotherapy.* New York: McGraw-Hill.

Lennox, N., Hyman, I. A., & Hughes. C. A. (1988). Institutionalization of a consultation-based service delivery system. In J. L. Graden, J. E. Zins, & M. E. Curtis (Eds.), *Alternative educational delivery systems: Enhancing instructional services for all students,* (pp. 71–89). Washington, DC: National Association of School Psychologists.

Lennox, N., Marks, E. S., Rodwin, H., Hughes, C., & Kaplan, H. (1986, April). *Dynamic, generic school consultation—Theory and practice.* Symposium presented at the annual convention of the National Association of School Psychologists, Ft. Lauderdale, FL.

Lewin, K. (1976). *Field theory as human science: Contributions of Lewin's Berlin group.* New York: Gardner Press.

Likert, R. (1961). *New patterns of management.* New York: McGraw-Hill.

Likert, R. (1967). *The human organization: Its management and value.* New York: McGraw-Hill.

Lippitt, G., & Lippitt, R. (1986). *The consulting process in action* (2nd ed.). LaJolla, CA: University Associates.

Litwin, G. H., & Stringer, Jr., R. A. (1968). *Motivation and organizational climate.* Boston: Harvard University. Division of Research.

Magary, J. (1967). Emerging viewpoints in school psychological services. In J. Magary (Ed.), *School psychological services,* (pp. 671–755). Englewood Cliffs, NJ: Prentice-Hall.

Maheady, L., Harper, G. F., Mallette, B., & Winstanley, N. (1991). Training and implementation requirements associated with the use of a class-wide peer tutoring system. *Education and Treatment of Children, 14*(3), 177–198.

Maher, C. A. (1986). Improving the instructional supervisory behavior of public school principals by means of time management: Experimental evaluation and social validation. *Professional School Psychology, 3,* 177–191.

Maher, C. A., & Bennett, R. W. (1984). *Planning and evaluation in special education services.* Englewood Cliffs, NJ: Prentice-Hall.

Maher, C. A., & Illback, R. J. (1985). Implementing school psychological service programs: Description and application of the DURABLE approach. *Journal of School Psychology, 23*(1), 81–89.

Maher, C. A., Illback, J. R., & Zins, J. E. (1984). Applying organizational psychology in schools: Perspectives and framework. In C. A. Maher, R. J. Illback, & J. E. Zins (Eds.), *Organizational psychology in the schools: A handbook for professionals* (pp. 5–20). Springfield, IL: C. C. Thomas.

Manz, C. C., & Sims, H. P. (1987). Leading workers to lead themselves: The external leadership of self-managing work teams. *Administrative Science Quarterly, 32,* 106–128.

Marks, E. S., & Rodwin, H. J. (1985, June). *The school psychologist-New roles: Whole school consultation.* Paper presented at the annual meeting of the Pennsylvania Psychological Association, Lancaster, PA.

Marks, E. S., Rodwin, H. J., & Weisenberg, J. (1987, June). *School consultation: Breaking the ice; handling the flood.* Paper presented at the annual meeting of the Pennsylvania Psychological Association, Lancaster, PA.

Marks, E. S., Rodwin, H. J., & Weisenberg, J. (1988, November). *Interdisciplinary approaches to whole school consultation.* Paper presented at the annual convention of the National Association of Social Workers, Philadelphia, PA.

Martens, B. K., Witt, J. C., Elliott, S. N., & Darveaux, D. X. (1985). Teacher judgments concerning the acceptability of school-based interventions. *Professional Psychology, 16,* 191–198.

Maslach, C. M., & Jackson, S. E. (1986). *The Maslach Burnout Inventory* (2nd ed.). Palo Alto, CA: Consulting Psychologists Press.

Maslow, A. H. (1970). *Motivation and personality* (2nd ed.). New York: Harper.

McKenzie, H. S. (1971). *Special education and consulting teachers.* Burlington, VT: Vermont State Department of Education.

McManus, M. E., & Kaufman, J. M. (1991). Working conditions of teachers of students with behavior disorders. *Behavioral Disorders, 16*(4), 247–259.

Medway, F. J. (1979). How effective is school consultation: A review of recent research. *Journal of School Psychology, 17*(3), 275–282.

Medway, F. J. (1982). School consultation research: Past trends & future directions. *Professional Psychology, 13,* 422–430.

Medway, F. J., & Cafferty, T. P. (1990). Contributions of social psychology to school psychology. In T. B. Gutkin & C. R. Reynolds (Eds.), *The handbook of school psychology* (pp. 175–197). New York: Wiley.

Merkel, W. T., & Carpenter, L. J. (1987). A cautionary note on the application of family therapy principles to organizational consultation. *American Journal of Orthopsychiatry, 57,* 111–115.

Meyers, J. (n.d.). *How teachers can maximize help from specialists in schools.* Unpublished manuscript, Department of School Psychology, Temple University, Philadephia.

Meyers, J. (1973). A consultation model for school psychological services. *Journal of School Psychology, 11,* 5–15.

Meyers, J. (1980, June). *Reactions to Spring Hill.* Paper presented at Spring Hill Symposium, National School Psychology Inservice Training Network, APA Division 16 and National Association of School Psychologists, Spring Hill, MN.

Meyers, J. (1989). The practice of psychology in the schools for the primary prevention of learning and adjustment problems in children. In L. A. Bond & B. E. Compas (Eds.), *Primary prevention and promotion in the schools* (pp. 391–422). Newbury Park, CA: Sage.

Meyers, J., Parsons, R. D., & Martin, R. (1979). *Mental health consultation in the schools.* San Francisco: Jossey-Bass.

Minor, M. W. (1972). Systems analysis and school psychology. *Journal of School Psychology, 10*(3), 227–232.

Minuchin, S. (1974). *Families and family therapy.* Cambridge, MA: Harvard University Press.

Moses, S. (1991a, July). Schools cannot easily buck student tracking. *APA Monitor,* p. 46.

Moses, S. (1991b, August). Researcher finds joy in helping kids learn. *APA Monitor,* p. 32.

Mowrer, O. H. (1972). Integrity groups: Basic principles and objectives. *Counseling Psychologist, 3*(2), 7–32.

Naglieri, J. A., LeBuffe, P. A., & Pfeiffer, S. I. (1992). *Devereux Behavior Rating Scale—School Form.* San Antonio, TX: Psychological Corporation.

National Education Association's Center for Innovation. (1992, April). *Survey Report.* Washington, DC: Author.

National Institute for Occupational Safety and Health. (1987). *Stress management in work settings* (DHHS Publication No. 87–111). Washington, DC: U.S. Government Printing Office.

Newman, R. (1967). *Psychological consultation in the schools.* New York: Basic Books.

Olympia, D., Jenson, W. R., Clark, E., & Sheridan, S. (1992). Training parents to facilitate homework completion: A model for home-school collaboration. In S. L. Christenson & J. C. Conoley (Eds.), *Home-School collaboration* (pp. 309–331). Silver Spring, MD: National Association of School Psychologists.

Parsons, R. D., & Meyers, J. (1984). *Developing consultation skills.* San Francisco: Jossey-Bass.

Pennsylvania Department of Education. (1988). *The school guide to needs assessment for improving student achievement.* Harrisburg, PA: Author.

Peter, L., & Hull, R. (1984). *The Peter principle.* New York: Bantam.

Phillips, B. N. (1981). Spring Hill revisited. *Professional Psychology, 12,* 288–290.

Piersal, W. C. (1985). Behavioral consultation: An approach to problem solving in educational settings. In J. R. Bergan (Ed.), *School psychology in contemporary society: An introduction* (pp. 252–280). Columbus, OH: C. Merrill.

Piersal, W. C., & Gutkin, T. B. (1983). Resistance to schoolbased consultation: A behavioral analysis of the problem. *Psychology in the Schools, 20,* 311–320.

Platt, H., & Bardon, J. (1967). The school psychologist's role with the mentally retarded. In J. Magary (Ed.), *School psychological services* (pp. 392–421). Englewood Cliffs, NJ: Prentice-Hall.

Poland, S. (1993, November). *Crisis intervention.* Program presentation at the meeting of the Association of School Psychologists of Pennsylvania, King of Prussia, PA.

Ponti, C. (1989). Pre-referral consultation and intervention. In A. Canter & P. Dawson (Eds.), *Directory of alternative service delivery models* (pp. 39–40). Washington, DC: National Association of School Psychologists.

Ponti, C. R., Zins, J. E., & Graden, J. L. (1988). Implementing a consultation-based delivery system to decrease referrals for special education: A case study. *School Psychology Review, 17*(1), 89–100.

Pryzwansky, W. B., & White, G. W. (1983). The influence of consultee characteristics on preferences for consultation approaches. *Professional Psychology, 14,* 457–461.

Pugach, M., & Johnson, L. J. (1989). Peer collaboration. In A. Canter & P. Dawson (Eds.), *Directory of alternative delivery service models* (pp. 45–46). Washington, DC: National Association of School Psychologists.

Pugach, M., & Johnson, L. J. (1990). Developing reflective teaching through structured dialogue. In R. T. Cliff, R. W. Houston, & M. C. Pugach (Eds.), *Encouraging reflective practice: An examination of issues and exemplars* (pp. 186–207). New York: Teachers College Press.

Rappaport, J. (1981). In praise of paradox: A social policy of empowerment over prevention. *American Journal of Community Psychology, 9,* 1–25.

Reddin, W. J. (1994). *Using tests to improve training.* Englewood Cliffs, NJ: Prentice-Hall.

Remer, R., Niguette, G. F., Anderson, G. L., & Terrell, J. E. (1984, September). A meta-system for the delivery of primary preventive interventions. *Journal of Counseling and Development, 63,* 30–34.

Rich, D. (1987). *Schools and families: Issues and actions.* Washington, DC: National Education Association.

Ritter, D. R. (1978). Effects of a school consultation program upon referral patterns of teachers. *Psychology in the Schools, 15,* 239–243.

Rogers, C. R. (1965). *Client-centered therapy: Its current practice.* Boston: Houghton-Mifflin.

Rosenfield, S. (1987). *Instructional consultation.* Hillsdale, NJ: Erlbaum.

Rosenfield, S. (1992). Developing school-based consultation teams: A design for organizational change. *School Psychology Quarterly, 7*(1), 27–46.

Rosenfield, S., & Shapiro, E. (1989, October). *Project LINK.* Symposium conducted at the annual Pennsylvania School Psychologists conference, University Park, PA.

Roth, W. (1980, June). *Conversion from referral to consultation model for delivery of psychological services.* Paper presented at the annual meeting of the Pennsylvania Psychological Association, Lancaster, PA.

Rutter, M., Maughan, B., Mortimer, P., & Ouston, J. (1979). *Fifteen thousand hours: Secondary schools and their effects on children.* Cambridge, MA: Harvard University Press.

Sagor, R. (1991). What Project LEARN reveals about collaborative action research. *Educational Leadership, 48*(6), 6–10.

Saper, B. (1982). Power to the psychologist. *Professional Psychology, 13,* 191–199.

Saporito, T., & Ross, E. (1987, June). *Consulting to management: An internal consulting vs. external consulting perspective.* Paper presented at the annual convention of the Pennsylvania Psychological Association, Lancaster, PA.

Sarason, S. (1982). *The culture of the school and the problem of change.* Boston: Allyn & Bacon.

Sarason, S. (1988, March). *Some personal reflections on school psychology.* Address to the 8th annual conference on the Future of Psychology in the Schools, Philadelphia, PA.

Sarason, S., Levine, M., Goldenberg, I., Cherlin, D., & Bennett, E. (1966). *Psychology in community settings.* New York: Wiley.

Schein, E. H. (1987). *Process consultation: Its role in organizational development.* Reading, MA: Addison-Wesley.

Scheinfeld, D. (1979). A design for renewing urban elementary schools. *Theory into Practice, 18*(2), 114–125.

Schmuck, R. A. (1982). Organizational development in the schools. In C. R. Reynolds & T. B. Gutkin (Eds.), *The handbook of school psychology* (pp. 829–857). New York: Wiley.

Schmuck, R. A. (1990). Organizational development in the schools. Contemporary concepts and practices. In T. B. Gutkin & C. R. Reynolds (Eds.), *The handbook of school psychology* (pp. 899–919). New York: Wiley.

Schroeder, C. S., & Miller, F. T. (1981). Entry patterns and strategies in consultation. In M. J. Curtis & J. E. Zins (Eds.), *The theory and practice of school consultation* (pp. 159–164). Springfield, IL: C. C. Thomas.

Schumm, J. S., & Vaughn, S. (1991). Making adaptations for mainstreamed students: General classroom teachers' perspectives. *RASE: Remedial and Special Education 12*(4), 18–27.

Sergiovanni, T. J., & Elliott, D. (1975). *Educational and organizational leadership in elementary schools.* Englewood Cliffs, NJ: Prentice-Hall.

Sergiovanni, T. J., & Starratt, R. J. (1988). *Supervision: Human perspectives.* New York: McGraw-Hill.

Shapiro, E. S. (1987). *Behavioral assessment in school.* Hillsdale, NJ: Erlbaum.

Shapiro, E. S., & Derr, T. F. (1990). Curriculum-based assessment. In T. B. Gutkin & C. R. Reynolds (Eds.), *The handbook of school psychology* (pp. 365–387). New York: Wiley,

Sheridan, S. (1991, December). Promoting home-school problem solving through conjoint behavioral consultation. *NASP Communique*, pp. 7–8.

Sheridan, S. (1993). Models for working with parents. In J. E. Zins, T. R. Kratochwill, & S. N. Elliott (Eds.), *The handbook of consultation services for children* (pp. 110–133). San Francisco: Jossey-Bass.

Sheridan, S., Kratochwill, T. R., & Elliott, S. N. (1990). Behavioral consultation with parents and teachers: Delivering treatment for socially withdrawn children at home and school. *School Psychology Review, 19*(1), 33–52.

Shore, K., & Vieland, C. (1989). And now for something completely different: The North Mercer family consultation center. *New Jersey Journal of School Psychology, 3,* 27–33.

Silverstein, J. (1989). Fostering parent-professional involvement in special education: A role for school psychology educators. *Trainer's Forum, 9*(2), 4–7.

Silverstein, J. (1991, June). IEP meetings often confusing to parents. *NASP Communique,* p. 6.

Simpson, R., & Poplin, M. (1981). Parents as agents of change. *School Psychology Review, 10,* 15–25.

Sindelar, P. T., Griffin, C. C., Smith, S. W., & Watanabe, A. K. (1992). Pre-referral intervention: Encouraging notes on preliminary findings. *Elementary School Journal, 92*(3), 245–259.

Singer, D. L., Whiton, M. B., & Fried, M. (1970). An alternative to traditional mental health services and consultation in schools: A social systems and group process approach. *Journal of School Psychology, 8*(3), 172–178.

Skinner, M. E. (1991). Facilitating parental participation during individualized education program conferences. *Journal of Educational and Psychological Consultation, 2*(3), 285–289.

Skinner, M. E., & Hales, M. R. (1992). Classroom teachers' explanations of student behavior: One possible barrier to the acceptance and use of applied behavior analysis procedures in the schools. *Journal of Educational and Psychological Consultation, 3*(3), 219–232.

Skrtic, T. M. (1991). The special education paradox: Equity on the way to excellence. *Harvard Educational Review, 61*(2), 148–206.

Slavin, R. E. (1990). *Cooperative learning.* Englewood Cliffs, NJ: Prentice-Hall.

Sleek, S. (1994, September). Psychology is finding a home in school-based health clinics. *APA Monitor, 25*(9), 1, 34.

Smelter, R., Bradley, W. R. & Yudewitz, G. J. (1994, September). Thinking of inclusion for all special needs students? Better think again. *Phi Delta Kappan, 76,* 35–38.

Smith, J. M., & Smith, D. E. P. (1976). *Child management: A program for parents and teachers.* Champaign, IL: Research Press.

Smith, J. S. (1993, August). *Leadership, vision and culture change.* Paper presented at the Pennsylvania Psychological Association workshop on Changing Organizational Culture, Carlisle, PA.

Smyth, J. (1989). Developing and sustaining critical reflection in teacher education. *Journal of Teacher Education, 40*(2), 2–9.

Snapp, M., Hickman, J. A., & Conoley, J. C. (1990). Systems interventions in school settings. In T. B. Gutkin & C. R. Reynolds (Eds.), *The handbook of school psychology* (pp. 920–934). New York: Wiley.

Sparks-Langer, G. M., & Berstein Colton, A. (1991). Synthesis of research on teachers' reflective thinking. *Educational Leadership, 48*(6), 37–44.

Stemmel, M. I., Abernathy, T. V., Butera, G., & Lesar, S. (1991). Teacher perceptions of the regular education initiative. *Exceptional Children, 58*(1). 9–24.

Stokes, S. (1982). *School-based staff support teams: A blue-print for action.* Reston, VA: Council for Exceptional Children.

Sundstrom, E., & Altman, I. (1989). Physical environments and working group effectiveness. In L. L. Cummings & B. Staw (Eds.), *Research in organizational behavior* (Vol. 11, pp. 175–209). Greenwich, CT: JAI Press.

Sundstrom, E., DeMeuse, K. P., & Futrell, D. (1990). Work teams: Applications and effectiveness. *American Psychologist, 45*(2), 120–133.

Tannenbaum, A., & Cooke, R. A. (1979). Organizational control: A review of studies using the Control Graph method. In C. J. Lammers & D. J. Hickson (Eds.), *Organizations alike and unlike* (pp. 183–210). London: Routledge & Kegan Paul.

Tharp, R. G. (1975). The triadic model of consultation: Current considerations. In C. A. Parker (Ed.), *Psychological consultation: Helping teachers meet special needs* (pp. 135–151). Reston, VA: University of Minnesota and the Council for Exceptional Children.

Tharp, R. G. & Wetzel, R. J. (1969). *Behavioral modification in the natural environment.* New York: Academic Press.

Thibaut, J. W., & Kelly, H. H. (1959). *The social psychology of groups.* New York: Wiley.

Thoresen, C. E., & Eagleston, J. R. (1985). Counseling for health. *Counseling Psychologist, 13*(1), 15–88.

Tice, C. (1987, January/February). Rescuing students. *NEA Today,* p. 10.

Tombari, M. L., & Bergan, J. R. (1978). Consultant cues and teacher verbalizations, judgments and expectations concerning children's adjustment problems. *Journal of School Psychology, 16,* 212–219.

Trachtman, G. (1981). On such a full sea. In *School Psychology Review, 10*(2), 138–181.

Tucker, J. (1981). The emperor's new clothes are hand-me-downs: Reaction to Baer & Bushnell. *School Psychology Review, 10*(2), 271–277.

Tuckman, B. W. (1965). Developmental sequence in small groups. *Psychological Bulletin, 63,* 384–389.

Tuckman, B. W., & Jensen, M. (1977). Stages of small group development revisited. *Group and Organizational Studies, 2,* 419–427.

Valentine, M. R. (1992). How to deal with difficult school discipline problems: A family systems approach adapted for schools. In S. L. Christenson & J. C. Conoley (Eds.), *Home-school collaboration* (pp. 357–382). Silver Spring, MD: National Association of School Psychologists.

Vanden Belt, A., & Peterson, C. (1991). Parental explanatory style and its relationship to the classroom performance of disabled and non-disabled children. *Cognitive Therapy and Research, 15*(4), 331–341.

Vinnicombe, S. (1980). *Secretaries, management and organizations.* London: Heinemann Educational Books.

Walberg, H. J. (1984). Families as partners in educational productivity. *Phi Delta Kappan, 65*(6), 397–400.

Wallin, J. E. W., & Ferguson, D. G. (1967). The development of school psychological services. In J. Magary (Ed.), *School psychological services* (pp. 1–29). Englewood Cliffs, NJ: Prentice-Hall.

Wedam, K. (1993). President's message. *New Jersey School Psychologist, 11*(4), 1.

Weiss, H. M., & Edwards, M. E. (1992). The family-school collaboration project: Systemic interventions for school improvement. In S. L. Christenson & J. C. Conoley (Eds.), *Home-school collaboration* (pp. 215–243). Silver Spring, MD: National Association of School Psychologists.

Weller, C., & Strawser, S. (1981). *Weller–Strawser Scales of Adaptive Behavior.* Novato, CA: Academic Therapy Publications.

Wellington, B. (1991). The promise of reflective practice. *Educational Leadership, 48*(6), 4–5.

West, J. F., & Cannon, G. S. (1988). Essential collaborative consultation competancies for regular and special education. *Journal of Learning Disability, 21*(1), 56–63.

West, J. F., & Idol, L. (1990). Collaborative consultation in the education of mildly handicapped and at-risk students. *RASE: Remedial and Special Education, 11*(1), 22–31.

West, J. F., Idol, L., & Cannon, G. (1987). *A curriculum for preservice and inservice preparation of classroom and special education teachers in collaborative consultation.* Austin, TX: University of Texas at Austin, Research and Training Project on School Consultation.

West, J. F., Idol, L., & Cannon, G. (1989). *Collaboration in the schools.* Austin, TX: Pro-Ed.

Whinnery, K. W., Fuchs, L. S., & Fuchs, D. (1991). General, special and remedial teachers' acceptance of behavioral and instructional strategies for mainstreaming students with mild handicaps. *RASE: Remedial and Special Education, 12*(4), 6–17.

White, R. W. (1958). Motivation reconsidered: The concept of competence. *Psychological Review, 66*(5), 297–333.

Whitworth, J. R., & Sutton, D. L. (1993). *WISC-III compilation.* Novato, CA: Academic Therapy Publications.

Wickstrom, K. F., & Witt, J. C. (1993). Resistance within school-based consultation. In J. E. Zins, T. R. Kratochwill, & S. N. Elliott (Eds.), *Handbook of consultation services for children* (pp. 159–178). San Francisco: Jossey-Bass.

Willower, D. J., Eidell, T. I., & Hoy, W. K. (1967). *The school and pupil control ideology* (Pennsylvania State University Studies No. 24). State College, PA: Pennsylvania State University.

Witt, J. C. (1986). Teachers' resistance to the use of schoolbased interventions. *Journal of School Psychology, 24,* 37–44.

Witt, J. C., & Elliott, S. N. (1985). Acceptability of classroom intervention strategies. In T. R. Kratochwill (Ed.), *Advances in school psychology* (Vol. IV, pp. 251–288). Hillsdale, NJ: Erlbaum.

Wrenn, G. (1967). Emerging viewpoints in school psychological services. In J. Magary (Ed.), *School psychological services* (pp. 671–755). Englewood Cliffs, NJ: Prentice-Hall.

Yanowitz, B. (1984). Improving our image: Effective public relations for school psychologists. *APA Division 16 Newsletter*, p. 6.

Ysseldyke, J. (1984, October). *Lookin' for LD in all the wrong places.* Paper presented at the Annual Pennsylvania School Psychologists Conference, University Park, PA.

Ysseldyke, J. E., Algozzine, B., & Allen, D. (1982). Participation of regular education teachers in special education team decision-making: A naturalistic investigation. *Exceptional Children 48*, 365–366.

Ysseldyke, J. E., Algozzine, B., & Mitchell, J. (1982). Special education team decision making: An analysis for current practice. *Personnel and Guidance Journal, 60*, 308–313.

Ysseldyke, J. E., & Christenson, S. L. (1986). *The Instructional Environment Scale.* Austin, TX: Pro-Ed.

Zigler, E., Kagan, S. L., & Muenchow, S. (1982). Preventive intervention in the schools. In C. R. Reynolds & T. B. Gutkin (Eds.), *The handbook of school psychology* (pp. 774–795). New York: Wiley.

Zins, J. E. (1981). Using data-based evaluation in developing school consultation services. In M. J. Curtis & J. E. Zins (Eds.), *The theory and practice of school consultation* (pp. 261–268). Springfield, IL: C. C. Thomas.

Zins, J. E. (1984). A scientific problem-solving approach to accountability procedures for school psychologists. *Professional Psychology: Research and Practice, 15*(1), 56–66.

Zins, J. E. (1992). Implementing school-based consultation services: An analysis of 5 years of practice. In R. K. Conyne & J. O'Neil (Eds.), *Organizational consultation: A casebook.* Newbury Park, CA: Sage.

Zins, J. E., Conyne, R. K., & Ponti, C. R. (1988). Primary prevention: Expanding the impact of psychological services in the schools. *School Psychology Review, 17*(4), 542–549.

Zins, J. E., & Curtis, M. J. (1984). Building consultation into the educational service delivery system. In C. A. Maher, R. J. Illback, & J. E. Zins (Eds.), *Organizational psychology in the schools: A handbook for professionals* (pp. 213–242). Springfield, IL: C. C. Thomas.

Zins, J. E., Curtis, M. J. Graden, J. L., & Ponti, C. R. (1988). *Helping students succeed in the regular classroom.* San Francisco: Jossey-Bass.

Zins. J. E., & Illback, R. J. (1993). Implementing consultation programs in child service systems. In J. E. Zins, T. R. Kratochwill, & S. N. Elliott (Eds.), *The handbook of consultation services for children* (pp. 204–226). San Francisco: Jossey-Bass.

Zins, J. E., & Ponti, C. R. (1990). Strategies to facilitate the implementation, organization and operation of system-wide consultation programs. *Journal of Educational and Psychological Consultation, 1*(3), 205–218.

Index